Medication in Maternity

Medication in Maternity
Infant Exposure and Maternal Information

Yvonne Brackbill, Ph.D.

Graduate Research Professor
Fellow, International Academy for Research
    in Learning Disabilities
Department of Psychology
University of Florida

Karen McManus

University of Florida

Lynn Woodward

University of Florida

International Academy for Research in Learning Disabilities
Monograph Series, Number 2

Ann Arbor   The University of Michigan Press

1992   1991   1990   1989   5   4   3   2

This research was supported in part by Maternal and Child Health
(Social Security, Title V) Grant MC-R-120455 from the Health
Resources and Services Administration.
   We gratefully acknowledge the assistance of Paul Doering,
Michael Ireson, James McClave, David Robinson, and Ronald
Stewart for their help. Thanks also to Mr. Harold Davis, Profes-
sional Affairs and Advisory Opinions, FDA, for his assistance in
obtaining information about specific drugs.

Library of Congress Cataloging in Publication Data

Brackbill, Yvonne.
   Medication in maternity.

   (International Academy for Research in Learning
Disabilities monograph series ; no. 2)
   Summaries in English, French, German, and Spanish.
   Bibliography: p.
   Includes index.
   1. Fetus—Effect of drugs on.   2. Central nervous
system—Effect of drugs on.   3. Pregnancy, Complications
of.   4. Drugs—Side effects.   5. Pregnant women—drug use.
6. Drugs—Information services—United States.   I. McManus,
Karen, 1957–   .   II. Woodward, Lynn.   III. Title.
IV. Series. [DNLM: 1. Drug Information Services—
utilization.   2. Drug Therapy—in pregnancy.   3. Fetus—
drug effects.   4. Infant, Newborn.   5. Learning Disorders
—chemically induced.   6. Labor—drug effects.
WQ 200 B797m]
RG627.6.D79B73   1985   618.3   85-1050
ISBN 0-472-08059-8 (pbk.)

Paperback ISBN : 978-0-472-08059-5

*This series of monographs published under the
sponsorship of the International Academy for
Research in Learning Disabilities is dedicated
to the recognition of Professor Alexander
Romanovich Luria, Ph.D., of the Union of Soviet
Socialist Republics, a world-class professional
whose work underscores a major development in
an understanding of the neurophysiological development of learning disabled children and adults.*

Contents

Abstract ix

Abstrakt xi

Résumé xv

Sumario xix

Preface xxiii

**Introduction: Drug Consumption, Infant Risk,
and Drug Information** 1

   Drug Consumption and Infant Risk   1

   Information: Prerequisite to Effective Health Decisions   2

Obstetrical Drugs as High-Tech Hazards 5

   Birth: High Risk Period for the Developing
   Central Nervous System   5

   Effects of Obstetric Drugs   6

   Summary and Conclusions   22

Medical Decision Making: Information as Power 25

   A Short History of Medical Disclosure   25

   Informed Consent: Moral Duty, Legal Mandate   27

   Respect for Autonomy: The Right to Be Informed   28

   Respect for Well-Being   31

The Florida Study 35

   Participants   35

   Sources of Data   38

   Interviewers   42

The Evidence 43
   Demographic Characteristics   43
   Health-Related Problems and Coping Strategies   46
   Drug-Taking Patterns during Pregnancy   51
   Patterns of Drug Administration during Childbirth   53
   Rx for Mothers Equals Risk for Babies?   57
   Mothers' Information about Drugs   82
   Individual Difference Variables   92

A Closer Look at the Findings 95
   Participant Profiles   96
   Health Problems and Risks   98
   Drug Remedies   99
   Drug Safety   101
   Mothers' Information about Drugs   109
   Summary   127

Appendixes 131
   A. Health-Promoting Behavior Items   133
   B. Maternal Drug Consumption: Drug Ingredients
   and Products Containing Those Ingredients   137
   C. Numbered References for Tables 14 and 15   143

References 167
Subject Index 183
Name Index 185

Abstract

The impetus for this study came from two bodies of empirical data, both of which are directly or indirectly related to learning disabilities. One is the large number of studies showing that administration of obstetric drugs is likely to produce behaviorally teratogenic effects. The second are those data showing that health care consumers, including pregnant women, want information about medications (as well as other aspects of health care); that they are ethically and legally entitled to such information; and that giving or withholding information and decision-making control can affect their physical and mental health.

The study itself investigated maternal drug consumption and infant drug exposure during pregnancy and childbirth, the status of those drugs with respect to adverse fetal effects, and the amount of information mothers have about the drugs they have consumed.

Participants were 602 mothers who delivered clinically normal babies. Of the total, 402 had chosen to deliver in-hospital ("Hospital Mothers"); 100, at a freestanding birth center ("Center Mothers"); and 100, at home ("Home Mothers").

Data on drug consumption and drug information were obtained by interview and from medical records. Drug information was scored according to consumer information standards recommended by the American Society of Hospital Pharmacists.

The three groups of mothers did not differ in the number of health-related problems they reported experiencing during their pregnancies. However, Hospital Mothers significantly exceeded Center and Home Mothers in resorting to drugs as the therapy of choice in coping with those problems. During pregnancy, Hospital and Center Mothers consumed significantly more prescription drugs, nonprescription drugs, and druglike products than did Home Mothers. During childbirth, significantly more drugs were administered to Hospital Mothers than to Center or Home Mothers.

Four approaches were used in assessing drug safety, defined as the absence of empirically demonstrated adverse fetal effects. First, inquiries revealed that most of the drugs actually administered during labor and delivery had never been approved for that purpose by FDA. Second, a literature search revealed no published reports of safety (or lack of it) for two-thirds of the prenatally consumed drug ingredients and one-third of the intrapartally administered drug ingredients. Third, for those drugs for which there are published reports, more than half of the drugs consumed or administered contain one or more ingredients implicated by empirical study as having adverse effects on the fetus. Fourth, a check of pharmacy shelves revealed that more than two-thirds of nonprescription products mothers reported consuming carried no labeled cautionary warning directed to pregnant women.

Apropos of drug information, the data indicated that, in general, mothers knew very little about the drugs they consumed during pregnancy and even less about the drugs administered to them during childbirth. Home Mothers were significantly better informed than Center Mothers, who, in turn, were significantly better informed than Hospital Mothers.

After exploring reasons for mothers' lack of knowledge about the drugs they consumed, the discussion extended to the role of informational gatekeeping in attaining and maintaining power; the relationship of gender to power and social influence; the rise of power in American medicine; and nondisclosure as an insitutional policy of the FDA.

Finally, it was noted that the variable most closely and consistently associated with drug consumption and drug information was choice of birthplace: hospital, freestanding birth center, or home.

Abstrakt

Der Anstoss fuer diese Untersuchung kam von 2 Gruppen empirischer Daten, von denen beide direkt oder indirekt eine Beziehung zu Lernunfaehigkeiten haben. Die eine davon ist eine grosse Gruppe von Untersuchungen, die zeigt, dass die Einnahme von geburtshilflichen Drogen wahrscheinlich "teratogenic" Verhaltensaenderungen bewirkt. Die zweite Gruppe besteht aus Daten, die zeigen, dass Patienten—schwangere Frauen eingeschlossen—Information ueber Drogen (und andere Aspekte der Gesundheitsfoerderung) verlangen; dass sie moralisch und juristisch zu solchen Informationen berechtigt sind; dass weiter das Geben oder Zurueckhalten solcher Information, sowie Entscheidungskontrolle deren organische und geistige Gesundheit beeinflussen kann.

Die Untersuchung selbst befasste sich mit dem muetterlichen Drogenkonsum und der Einwirkung auf das Kind waehrend der Schwangerschaft und der Geburt, der negativen Einwirkung solcher Drogen auf den Foetus und der Menge von Information die Muetter ueber Drogen haben, die sie eingenommen haben.

Teilnehmer waren 602 Muetter, die klinisch normale Kinder zur Welt brachten. Davon hatten 402 im Krankenhaus entbunden ("Hospital Mothers"); 100 in einem freien Geburtszentrum ("Center Mothers"); und 100 zu Hause ("Home Mothers").

Daten ueber Drogenkonsum und Drogeninformation wurde durch Befragen und aus Krankengeschichten erhalten. Die Drogeninformation wurde in Uebereinstimmung mit Konsumer-Informationsnormen gemacht, die von der American Society of Hospital Pharmacists empfohlen weren.

Die Zahl der gesundheitlichen Probleme, die die Muetter waehrend ihrer Schwangerschaft hatten, waren dieselben in den drei Gruppen. Allerdings nahmen "Hospital Mothers" wesentlich mehr Drogen ein um mit diesen Problemen fertig zu werden. Waehrend der Schwangerschaft nahmen "Hospital" und "Center Mothers" wesentlich mehr apothekenpflichtige Drogen, nicht-apothekenpflichtige Drogen und Drogenaehnliche Produkte ein wie "Home Mothers." Waehrend der Geburt empfingen "Hospital Mothers" wesentlich mehr Drogen wie "Center" oder "Home Mothers."

Die Unschaedlichkeit der Drogen, wobei Unschaedlichkeit als Abwesenheit empirisch nachweisbarer negativer Effekte auf den Foetus definiert wurde, wurde auf vier verschiedene Arten untersucht. Erstens: Nachfragen zeigten, dass die Mehrheit der Drogen, die waehrend der Geburtswehen und der Geburt gegeben wurden, nie von der Food and Drug Administration (FDA) fuer diesen Zweck genehmigt waren. Zweitens: In der Literatur waren keine veroeffentlichten Berichte ueber die gesundheitliche Vertraeglichkeit (oder negativen Wirkungen) von zwei Drittel der Drogenbestandteile, die vor der Geburt eingenommen wurden, und ein Drittel der Drogenbestandteile, die waehrend der Geburt verabreicht wurden, zu finden. Drittens: Bei Drogen, fuer die veroeffentlichte Berichte bestehen, hatten mehr als die Haelfte der konsumierten oder verabreichten Drogen einen oder mehr Bestandteile, die auf Grund der empirischen Befunde einen negativen Einfluss auf den Foetus hatten. Viertens: Eine Kontrolle der Apothekenvorraete zeigte, dass mehr als zwei Drittel der nicht-apothekenpflichtigen Produkte, die von Muettern eingenommen wurden, keine Warnungsaufschriften trugen in Bezug auf schwangere Frauen.

A propos, Drogeninformation: Die Daten zeigen, dass die Muetter im Allgemeinen sehr wenig ueber die Drogen wussten, die sie waehrend der Schwangerschaft eingenommen hatten und noch weniger ueber die Drogen, die ihnen waehrend der Geburt berabreicht wurden. "Home Mothers" waren wesentlich besser informiert als "Center Mothers" und diese wiederum wesentlich besser als "Hospital Mothers."

Nach Erforschung der Gruende fuer die Unwissenheit der Muetter in Bezug auf Drogen, die sie einnahmen, befasste sich die Diskussion weiterhin mit der Rolle, die die "informational gatekeeping" (Kontrolle) in Bezug auf Erreichung und Aufrechterhaltung von Macht spielt; der Beziehung von Geschlecht zu Macht und gesellschaftlicher Einfluss; dem Anstieg der Macht in der amerikanischen Medizin; der Verschwiegenheit als Satzungsregel der FDA.

Endlich wurde beobachtet, dass der Variabilitaetsfaktor, am engsten und konsistent mit dem Drogenkonsum und mit der Drogeninformation verbunden, war die Wahl des Entbindungsplatzes: Krankenhaus, freies Geburtszentrum oder eigenes Heim.

Résumé

Cette étude ressort de deux ensembles de données empiriques ayant des rapports directs ou bien indirects avec les troubles d'apprentissage. Un ensemble de données porte sur le grand nombre d'études démontrant que l'administration de médicaments obstétriques peut provoquer des effets tératogéniques dans le comportement. L'autre ensemble se rapporte aux données démontrant que les usagers du service médical, y compris les femmes enceintes, demandent à être informés des médicaments qu'elles consomment (ainsi que des autres aspects du service médical); que d'un point de vue légal et moral ces usagers ont droit à cette information; et que la disponibilité de cette information et la responsabilité des décisions à cet égard peuvent mettre en cause leur psychisme et leur pathologie.

L'étude elle-même porte sur la consommation de médicaments par les femmes enceintes et sur le degré d'exposition de l'enfant à ces médicaments pendant la grossesse et l'accouchement. Elle examine aussi le status actuel de ces médicaments et leurs effets adverses sur le foetus, ainsi que l'accessibilité de cette information aux futures mères.

602 femmes accouchées d'enfants cliniquement normaux ont participé à cette enquête. Sur le total, 402 femmes ont préféré accoucher à l'hôpital ("accouchées à l'hôpital"); 100 en maternité ("accouchées en maternité"); et 100 à domicile ("accouchées à domicile").

Les données portant sur l'information et sur la consommation de médicaments ont été obtenues à l'aide d'interviews et de dossiers médicaux. L'information sur les médicaments a été enregistrée selon les standards recommendés par l'Association des Pharmacistes Hospitaliers Américains.

Le nombre de problèmes enregistrés chez les femmes pendant la grossesse est resté constant pour les trois groupes d'accouchées. Cependant, le nombre d'accouchées à l'hôpital ayant eu recours aux médicaments dépasse largement celui des accouchées en maternité et à domicile. Chez les accouchées à l'hôpital et en maternité la consommation de produits pharmaceutiques sous ordonnance ou en vente libre est supérieure à celle des accouchées à domicile. Le taux de médicaments administrés pendant l'accouchement est nettement plus élevé à l'hôpital qu'en maternité ou à domicile.

Quatre méthodes ont servi à établir l'innocuité des médicaments (l'innocuité se définissant par l'absence d'effets adverses—empiriquement démontrés—sur le foetus). Premièrement, l'enquête a révélé que la plupart des médicaments administrés pendant les douleurs et pendant l'accouchement n'avaient jamais été approuvés pour cet usage par la Food and Drug Administration (FDA). Deuxièmement, les recherches effectuées dans la littérature médicale n'ont révélé aucune étude publiée sur les dangers possibles pour les deux tiers des médicaments consommés pendant la période prénatale et pour un tiers des médicaments administrés pendant l'accouchement. Troisièmement, plus de la moitié des médicaments faisant l'objet de rapports publiés contiennent un ou plusieurs ingrédients reconnus par des études empiriques comme provoquant des effets adverses sur le foetus. Quatrièmement, un contrôle dans les pharmacies a révélé que plus des deux tiers des produits pharmaceutiques en vente libre ne comportaient aucune contre-indication pour les femmes enceintes.

Les données portant sur l'information indiquent que les accouchées étaient, en général, très peu informées des médicaments consommés pendant leur grossesse et l'étaient encore moins en ce qui concerne les médicaments administrés pendant l'accouchement. Les accouchées à domicile semblaient être les mieux informées par rapport aux accouchées en maternité et à l'hôpital respectivement.

Après avoir exploré les raisons d'un tel manque d'information, le débat s'est porté sur le rôle joué par le "gatekeeping" (contrôle) en matière d'information concernant l'obtention et le maintien du pouvoir; sur les rapports du sexe au pouvoir et à l'influence sociale; sur la montée en puissance de la médcine américaine; et sur la politique systématique de non-divulgation pratiquée par la FDA.

Enfin, il a été noté que le choix du lieu d'accouchement—l'hôpital, la maternité ou le domicile—reste la variable la plus étroitement et logiquement liée à l'information et à la consommation de médicaments.

Sumario

El impetu para este estudio resultó de dos cuerpos de datos empíricos, ambos teniendo directa o indirecta relación a dishabilidades para aprender. Uno consiste de la multitud de estudios demostrando que la administración de drogas obstetricas probablemente producen efectos *teratogenic* de la conducta. El segundo consiste de esos datos demostrando que consumidores de cuidados de salud, incluyendo mujeres embarazadas, quieren información sobre drogas (y otros aspectos de cuidados de salud); que moralmente y legalmente tienen derecho a tal información; y que dando o negando información y control sobre decisiónes puede afectar su salud física y mental.

El estudio investigó el uso maternal de drogas y la exposición a drogas de infantes durante el embarazo y el parto, el estado de esas drogas respecto a efectos adversos a el feto, y la cantidad de información que tienen las madres sobre las drogas que han consumido.

Participantes fueron 602 madres que dieron parto a niños clinicamente normales. De ese total, 402 escogieron dar parto en un hospital ("Madres de Hospital"); 100 en un Centro de Nacimiento ("Madres de Centros"); y 100 en el hogar ("Madres de Hogar").

Datos sobre el consumo de drogas y información sobre drogas fueron obtenidos de entrevistas y de datos en historias médicas. Informaciónes sobre drogas fueron apuntadas segun los estandares de información al consumidor recomendados por la Sociedad Americana de Farmacéuticos de Hospitales.

Los tres grupos de madres no demostraron diferencias en el número de problemas relacionados a salud que reportaron experienciar durante el embarazo. Sin embargo, Madres de Hospital excedieron significamente a las Madres de Centros y de Hogar en recurrir a drogas como terapia de preferencia para lidiar con esos problemas. Durante el embarazo, Madres de Hospital y de Centros consumieron significamente mas drogas de receta, drogas sin recetas, y productos parecidos a drogas que las Madres de Hogar. Durante el parto, significamente mas drogas fueron administradas a Madres de Hospital que a las Madres de Centros o Hogar.

Cuatro modos de proceder fueron utilizados en determinar la seguridad de drogas, definido como la ausencia de empiricamente demostradas reacciones adversas al feto. Primero, averiguaciónes revelaron que casi todas las drogas administradas durante el parto no habian sido aprobadas para ese propósito por el Food and Drug Administration (FDA). Segundo, una examinación de la literatura reveló ningunos reportes publicados (o la ausencia de tal reportes) para dos terceras partes de los ingredientes consumidos prenatalmente y una tercera parte de los ingredientes consumidos durante el parto. Tercero, para esas drogas donde sí existen reportes publicados, mas de la mitad de las drogas consumidas o administradas contienen uno o mas ingredientes que han sido implicados por estudios empiricos de tener reacciones adversas para el feto. Cuarto, una examinación de farmacias revelo mas de dos terceras partes de productos sin receta que madres reportaron consumir no llevaban una etiqueta de precaución dirigida a mujeres embarazadas.

A propósito de informacioń sobre drogas, los datos indican que, generalmente, madres conocian muy poco de las drogas que estaban tomando durante el embarazo y menos sobre las drogas administradas durante el parto. Madres de Hogar estaban significamente mejor informadas que las Madres de Centros, y ellas en turno estaban significamente mejor informadas que Madres de Hospital.

Despues de examinar razones por la falta de conocimiento de madres sobre drogas que ellas consumen, la discusión se extendió a el papel que desempeña el "portero informaciónal" en conseguir y sostener el poder; la relación de género al poder, y a la influencia social; la elevación de poder de la medicina Americana; y la falta de revelación como politica institucional del FDA.

Finalmente, fue notado que el variable mas cercano y consistentemente asociado con el consumo de drogas y información sobre drogas fue la selección de lugar de nacimiento: un hospital, un centro de nacimiento, o el hogar.

Preface

The estimated prevalence of American children in need of special education has been put at 10 to 15 percent (Gaddes 1980, 17). The seriousness of this problem is reflected in the considerable number of articles bearing on learning disorders and related dysfunctions that have appeared in the research literature over the last several decades (Hallahan and Cruickshank 1973, 156).

Despite the concern over learning disorders, very little of the research devoted to it has focused on its primary causes. To illustrate, in the decade between 1971 and 1980, PsyINFO Retrospective (1982) lists "etiology" as a major descriptor term for only .03 percent of original research studies in learning disorders. In the recent Torgesen and Dice review of the characteristics of research on learning disabilities, "etiology" is absent altogether from the classification of studies by major content area (1980, 532). What accounts for the paucity of research into the causes of such an important problem as learning disorders?

One major reason for the shortfall of etiologically oriented research is the long temporal lag between the identification of a learning disorder (LD)—the median age of LD research subjects is about ten years (Torgesen and Dice 1980, 533, table 2)—and the events during prenatal, perinatal, or early postnatal life that may have contributed to that problem. It is difficult to establish cause-effect relationships through retrospective studies but even more difficult to fund and carry out prospective studies of ten years' duration.

Another reason for the lack of etiological research stems

from the drastic behavioral metamorphosis that occurs during the first years of life and the consequent difficulty in identifying in infancy the behavioral precursors of later LD that would allow us to predict the occurrence, nature, and extent of that dysfunctional state. The presence of a learning disorder in an older child is inferred from dysfunctions in the perceptual, cognitive, and motor components of such skills as reading and writing. But infants cannot read or write. Their perceptual, cognitive, and motor behaviors are either undeveloped, extremely restricted, or qualitatively different from those characterizing the older child.

Another factor discouraging etiological research into learning disorders is that whatever the nature of the neurophysiological aberrations underlying the behavioral manifestations of LD, they are probably neither homogeneous nor unique. Even worse, they are likely to be aberrations of a subtle or low-level nature, difficult to measure or, indeed, even to detect, given our current technologies. (See Vorhees, Brunner, and Butcher 1979.)

Still another reason for the research hiatus into primary causes of learning disorders is the emphasis by some workers on treatment rather than prevention, along with their belief that knowledge about causal factors contributes nothing to knowledge about effective treatment. (See discussion by Ross and Ross 1982, 64.) As Cruickshank has commented, many investigators fail to see the importance of neurons for spelling (1980, vi).

Nevertheless, both logical considerations and empirical evidence compel us to acknowledge that perceptual and cognitive processes are mediated by neurophysiological processes and that dysfunction in these neurophysiological processes leads to dysfunction in the perceptual and cognitive behaviors they mediate, including those dysfunctions we term *learning disorders*. One certain cause of early dysfunction—and a probable cause of later dysfunction—are some of the drugs to which the central nervous system may be exposed during the period when it

is developing most rapidly and is therefore maximally vulnerable to the effects of teratogenic and toxic agents.[1] Although
the first half of the Introduction is devoted to reviewing some
of this evidence, our research was not primarily concerned
with the contribution of adverse drug effects to learning disorders or other behavioral dysfunction. Rather, the research
went beyond this and asked, what is the contribution to dysfunctional behavior from the consumption of teratogenic and
toxic drugs? Since drugs have such potential for teratogenic
damage to fetus and newborn, why do pregnant mothers consume them? Do they lack information about these adverse side
effects? Why? What are the roadblocks to information? What
motives spur the gatekeepers of information to withhold or
disperse it?

---

1. A teratogenic agent is defined as one capable of producing anatomical,
physiological, or behavioral changes when administered to an organism during
prenatal, perinatal, or early postnatal periods of morphological and central
nervous system development. A toxic agent is defined as one causing disturbance of bodily function, damage to body, impairment of health, or destruc-
tion of life.

Introduction: Drug Consumption, Infant Risk, and Drug Information

Drug Consumption and Infant Risk

Medications or drugs[2] are the most widely used form of health care intervention in the United States. Among the major users of drugs are pregnant and parturient women. For example, Doering and Stewart (1978) found that, on the average, women consume eleven different drugs during the nine-month prenatal period and are exposed to seven different drugs during labor and delivery. Maternal drug consumption during these periods can have serious consequences for the unborn child.

Prenatal and early postnatal periods are periods of maximum vulnerability to adverse structural and functional effects of drugs and other teratogens.[3] The developing human is most vulnerable to structural teratogenesis during the first three months of pregnancy. However, the high-risk period for behavioral teratogenesis is much longer, lasting from just after conception to about eighteen months after birth.

2. Drugs, as defined by federal statute, are (1) articles intended for use in the diagnosis, cure, mitigation, treatment, or prevention of disease in man or other animals; and (2) articles other than food intended to affect the structures or any function of the body of man or other animals. (*A Legislative History of the Federal Food, Drug, and Cosmetic Act and Its Amendments*. Vols. 1–24. Washington, D.C.: General Printing Office, 1979.)

3. A teratogen is any agent capable of producing anatomical, physiological, or behavioral changes when administered to an organism during prenatal, perinatal, or early postnatal periods of morphological and central nervous system development.

Some drugs are known or documented teratogens. Others are suspected teratogens. Many have yet to be studied with respect to teratogenicity. Drugs that can be taken safely before pregnancy may be quite harmful to the developing child if taken during pregnancy. For example, Americans consume aspirin, a known teratogen, at the rate of 1,500 pounds per hour.[4] How many pregnant women are among these consumers? To what other drugs are their unborn children incidentally exposed during pregnancy and childbirth and how safe are those drugs? Two main purposes of this study were to investigate drug consumption during pregnancy and childbirth and to assess the safety for the unborn child of the drugs to which it is exposed.

Information: Prerequisite to Effective Health Decisions

Every year seven million American women and men become mothers and fathers. More than three million of their babies are born in hospitals, under obstetrical practices referred to by physicians and consumers alike as aggressively interventionistic (Brackbill, Rice, and Young 1984). Chief among these interventions is the obstetrician's heavy reliance on drugs, both for vaginal delivery and surgical delivery (now estimated to exceed 20 percent of all births for the nation as a whole).

American mothers and fathers, among other health care consumers, have become increasingly concerned with getting information about drugs and about other matters relating to their own health and the health of their children. Their concerns include the following:

- Health care consumers want information about the general status of their health.

---

4. Drug Information Service, College of Pharmacy, University of Florida, Gainesville, Florida, 1983.

- They want information about the nature and probable course of their own health problems.
- They want information about the benefits and risks of proposed treatments, including drugs.
- They want information about alternative forms of treatment.
- They want to share in the decision-making process in any matter pertaining to their own health or that of their children.

In support of their demands, health care consumers point to a variety of ethical, legal, and scientific reasons why they are entitled to health information and shared decision making.

- Providing health information and the opportunity to share in decision making constitute ethical obligations of health fiduciaries toward their patients.
- Information and shared decision making are now guaranteed by the legal doctrine of informed consent.
- Research shows that having information and decision-making control actually improves mental and physical health while withholding information and denying control actually impairs health.
- Providing health information is the official policy of all major professional organizations in the health industry.

But are consumers really getting information and sharing in decisions affecting their own health? This question was the mandated focus of attention recently by the President's Commission for the Study of Ethical Problems in Medicine and Biomedical and Behavioral Research (1982). The same question was also central to the present investigation, in which we asked to what extent mothers, as health care consumers, actually have information and decision-making control with respect to the drugs they consume during pregnancy and delivery.

CHAPTER 1

Obstetrical Drugs as High-Tech Hazards

Birth: High Risk Period for the Developing
Central Nervous System

During prenatal and early postnatal life, maximal vulnerability to teratogenic insult occurs during periods of rapid growth and development. The developing human is most susceptible to structural impairment during the first three months of pregnancy when the organs and the skeletal system are developing most rapidly. In contrast to the skeletal system and other major organs, the central nervous system (CNS) has a much longer period of rapid development, beginning just after conception and lasting until about eighteen months after birth. Therefore, it has a much longer period of susceptibility to teratogenic insult.

Since, by the time of birth, the skeletal system and most major organs are well beyond their period of most rapid development, drugs and other teratogens do not pose the threat of structural defect that they posed earlier. The CNS, however, is still developing rapidly at this time. Drugs administered during childbirth may alter the neurobehavioral functions mediated by the still developing CNS as well as the microstructures underlying those functions. (See Wilson's 1977 discussion of the progression from organogenesis to histogenesis to functional maturation.)

Vulnerability to drugs and other teratogens at birth is increased by the immaturity of the fetus. Most drugs and drug metabolites cross the placenta and readily enter the fetal circulation. Once in the circulation, drugs are drawn to highly perfused organs (e.g., the brain, liver, and kidneys) and tend to accumulate there in much greater concentrations than they would in the mature organism. The immature blood-brain barrier allows drugs and drug metabolites to pass through and lodge in the brain. Clearance of these toxic substances from the brain and other organs takes much longer than in the mature organism because drug metabolism and excretion is impaired by immature liver and kidney function.

The vulnerability of the rapidly developing CNS, coupled with the functional immaturity of the fetus at the time of birth, creates a situation in which impairment can follow a single drug administration. Contrary to popular, intuitively based belief, chronic administration is not necessary for behavioral teratogenesis to occur. (However, this is not to deny that repeated chronic administration may result in more marked or extensive damage than acute administration.)

There are a number of published research studies that have examined the behavioral effects of obstetric medication on the infant. (*Behavioral effect* will be used synonymously with *neurobehavioral effect*.) These studies will now be described and summarized.

Effects of Obstetric Drugs

Overview of the Studies

There are currently fifty-nine published studies which have examined the behavioral effects of obstetric medication. The findings of these studies are summarized in table 1. In evaluating these findings, we have defined significance as statistically significant effects ($p < .05$) for 50 percent or more of the measures of a particular behavioral variable at one or more of the ages at which that behavior was measured. Nonsignificance means no statistically significant effects ($p > .05$) for more than 50 percent of the measures of a particular behavioral variable at all the ages measured.

TABLE 1. Summary of Published Research Studies Examining the Effects of Obstetric Medication on Infant Behavior

Study	Type of Obstetric Medication[1]	Behavioral Variables[2]										Comments
		Motor	Habituation	Orientation	Reflex	Autonomic Regulation	Range of State	Regulation of State	Feeding	Social Interaction	EEG	
1. Abboud et al. 1982	Local	NS	NS	NS	NS		NS	NS	NS (see Reflex)			
2. Aleksandrowicz and Aleksandrowicz 1974	Mixed	NS	Sig	NS	NS	NS	NS	NS				See critique by Federman and Yang 1976
3. Baraka et al. 1981	Mixed	NS	NS	NS	NS				NS (see Reflex)			
4. Baraka et al. 1982	Mixed	NS	NS	NS	NS				NS (see Reflex)			
5. Belsey et al. 1981	Pre-An	Sig	NS	Sig			Sig	Sig		Sig		
6. Bonta et al. 1979	Pre-An	NS	NS	Sig	NS							Sig Scanlon general assessment 4, 24 hrs. Sig Scanlon test score 24 hrs. (NS 1, 4 hrs.)

[1]Genl = general anesthesia; Local = local anesthesia; Pre-An = preanesthetic medication; Mixed = some combination of the above.

[2]Sig = significant ($p \leq .05$); NS = nonsignificant ($p > .05$). For a complete definition of significance and nonsignificance, see p. 6 in the text. Superscript letters refer to notes in Comments column.

TABLE 1—Continued

Study	Type of Obstetric Medication[1]	Motor	Habituation	Orientation	Reflex	Autonomic Regulation	Range of State	Regulation of State	Feeding	Social Interaction	EEG	Comments
7. Borgstedt and Rosen 1968	Pre-An										Sig	
8. Brackbill et al. 1974a	Pre-An	Sig	Sig	Sig	Sig	Sig	Sig	Sig				Sig total score Brazelton test
9. Brackbill et al. 1974b	Pre-An		Sig									
10. Brackbill 1976	Mixed		Sig[a]									[a] $p < .10$
11. Brazelton 1961	Pre-An								Sig[a]	Sig (see Feeding)		[a]Sig responsiveness to feeding days 1–4 (NS days 5, 6)
12. Brazelton et al. 1979	Mixed	Sig	Sig	Sig		Sig	Sig	NS				
13. Brower et al. 1978	Pre-An			Sig							Sig[a]	[a]Sig with auditory stimulation only
14. Brown et al. 1975	Pre-An								NS	NS (see Feeding)		
15. Busacca et al. 1982	Pre-An	NS	NS	NS	NS	NS	NS					
16. Clark et al. 1976	Pre-An											Sig total score modified Scanlon test (individual items not analyzed)

Study	Anesthesia					Reflex	Notes
17. Conway and Brackbill 1970	Mixed	Sig	Sig[a]	Sig		NS (see Reflex)	[a]Sig day 5 (NS day 2) Sig total score on Graham Scale
18. Corke 1977	Pre-An	Sig	Sig	NS	Sig		Sig total Scanlon test NS Scanlon test score
19. Datta et al. 1980	Local						
20. Dubignon et al. 1969	Mixed					Sig[a]	[a]Sig nutritive sucking (NS nonnutritive sucking)
21. Emde et al. 1975	Mixed				Sig		
22. Friedman et al. 1978	Mixed		Sig	NS	NS		
23. Hodgkinson et al. 1976	1 Genl 2 Pre-An	1 Sig 2 NS	1 Sig 2 NS	1 Sig 2 Sig	1 Sig 2 NS	1 Sig 2 Sig[a] (see Reflex)	[a]Sig rooting (NS sucking) 1 Sig Scanlon general assessment 2 Sig Scanlon general assessment
24. Hodgkinson et al. 1977	Genl	Sig	Sig[a]	Sig	Sig	Sig (see Reflex)	[a]Sig day 1 (NS day 2) Sig Scanlon general assessment
25. Hodgkinson et al. 1978a	Pre-An	Sig[a]	Sig	Sig	Sig	Sig (see Reflex)	[a]Sig 2, 4 hrs. (NS 24 hrs.) Sig Scanlon general assessment
26. Hodgkinson et al. 1978b	Genl	Sig[a]	Sig	Sig	Sig[a]	Sig (see Reflex)	[a]Sig day 1 (NS day 2) [b]Sig day 1 (NS day 2) Sig Scanlon general assessment

TABLE 1—*Continued*

Study	Type of Obstetric Medication[1]	Behavioral Variables[2]										Comments
		Motor	Habituation	Orientation	Reflex	Autonomic Regulation	Range of State	Regulation of State	Feeding	Social Interaction	EEG	
27. Hodgkinson et al. 1978c	1 Pre-An 2 Genl	1 Sig 2 Sig[a]	1 Sig 2 Sig	1 Sig 2 Sig	1 Sig 2 Sig							[a]Sig day 2 (NS day 1) 1 Sig Scanlon general assessment 2 Sig Scanlon general assessment
28. Hollmen et al. 1978	Local	NS			Sig[a]				Sig (see Reflex)			[a]Sig 2, 4, 8 hrs. and days 1, 2 (NS days 3, 4, 7)
29. Horowitz et al. 1977	Mixed	Sig		Sig			Sig	Sig				
30. Hughes et al. 1948	Pre-An					NS					Sig	
31. Hughes et al. 1950	Pre-An										Sig	
32. Kraemer et al. 1972	Mixed								Sig			
33. Kron et al. 1966	Pre-An								Sig			
34. Lieberman et al. 1979	1 Local 2 Pre-An	1 NS 2 NS	1 NS 2 NS	1 NS 2 NS			1 NS 2 NS	1 NS 2 NS		1 Sig 2 NS		

10

Study									NS Scanlon test score
35. Lund et al. 1977	Local								
36. McGuinness et al. 1978	Local	Sig	NS	NS	NS				
37. Meis et al. 1978	Local	Sig[a]	NS	NS	Sig[b]	Sig[c]		Sig (see Reflex)	[a]Sig 2, 24 hrs. (NS 6 hrs.) [b]Sig 6 hrs. (NS 2, 24 hrs.) [c]Sig 6, 24 hrs. (NS 2 hrs.)
38. Merkow et al. 1980	Local	NS		NS	NS				
39. Moreau and Birch 1974	Genl		Sig	NS	NS				
40. Murray et al. 1981	Local	Sig[a]			Sig[b]	Sig[c]	Sig[d]	Sig[e] Sig	[a]Sig day 1 (NS day 5 or 1 month) [b]Sig when mother tested (NS when experimenter tested) [c]Sig day 1 (NS day 5 or 1 month) [d]Sig day 1, 5; Sig 1 month when mother tested (NS when experimenter tested) [e]Sig feeding as measured by home diary (NS when feeding observed by experimenter) Sig total Brazelton test score

11

TABLE 1—*Continued*

Study	Type of Obstetric Medication[1]	Behavioral Variables[2]										Comments
		Motor	Habituation	Orientation	Reflex	Autonomic Regulation	Range of State	Regulation of State	Feeding	Social Interaction	EEG	
41. Nesheim et al. 1979	Local	NS	Sig	NS	NS							
42. Ounsted et al. 1978	Mixed	NS		NS	NS							
43. Palahniuk et al. 1977	Mixed	Sig[a]	NS	Sig	NS							[a]Sig 6 hrs. (NS 24 hrs.) NS Scanlon general assessment
44. Parke et al. 1972	Mixed									NS		
45. Richards and Bernal 1972	Pre-An								Sig[a]	Sig (see Feeding)		[a]Sig feeding behavior (NS nonnutritive sucking)
46. Rooth et al. 1983	Local						Sig					
47. Rosenblatt et al. 1981	Local	Sig		Sig		Sig	Sig[a]	Sig[b]				[a]Sig days 1, 3, 21, 42 (NS day 7) [b]Sig days 3 and 42 (NS days 1, 7, 21)

12

Study	Type								Reflex	Notes
48. Scanlon et al. 1974	Local	Sig	Sig[a]	NS	Sig[b]				Sig[c] (see Reflex)	[a]Sig 2, 4, 6 hrs. (NS 8 hrs.) [b]Sig 4, 6, 8 hrs. (NS 2 hrs.) [c]Sig rooting (NS sucking)
49. Scanlon et al. 1976	Local	NS	NS	NS	NS				NS (see Reflex)	NS Scanlon test score
50. Shnider et al. 1979	Genl									
51. Standley et al. 1974	Mixed	Sig		NS		Sig	Sig			
52. Stechler 1964	Pre-An			Sig						
53. Stefani et al. 1982	Mixed	NS	NS	NS	NS		NS		NS (see Reflex)	
54. Tronick et al. 1976	Mixed	Sig[a]	NS	NS	NS	NS	NS	Sig[b]	NS (see Reflex)	[a]Sig 12 hrs. (NS days 2, 3, 4, 5, 7, 10) [b]Sig day 10 (NS days 1, 2, 3, 4, 5, 7)

TABLE 1—Continued

Study	Type of Obstetric Medication[1]	Behavioral Variables[2]										Comments
		Motor	Habituation	Orientation	Reflex	Autonomic Regulation	Range of State	Regulation of State	Feeding	Social Interaction	EEG	
55. VanderMaelen et al. 1975	Mixed		Sig[a]				NS					[a]Sig 4, 8, 12, 48 hrs. (NS .5, 24 hrs.)
56. Wiener et al. 1979	1 Pre-An 2 Local 3 Mixed	1 NS 2 Sig 3 NS	1 Sig[a] 2 NS 3 NS		1 NS 2 NS 3 Sig				1 NS 2 NS 3 Sig (see Reflex)			[a]Sig at 4, 8, 12, 48 hrs. (NS .5, 24 hrs.)
57. Woodson and DaCosta-Woodson 1980	Pre-An			NS			Sig	Sig				
58. Writer et al. 1981	Pre-An	NS	NS	NS	NS							
59. Yang et al. 1976	Mixed		Sig				Sig		NS			

14

Almost all published studies of obstetric medication and infant behavior have been carried out on infants six weeks of age and younger. Only three of the fifty-nine studies have tested for behavioral effects beyond this age (table 1, refs. 10, 22, 42). No studies have tested for effects of obstetric medication on behavior beyond twelve months of age.

The outcome of the fifty-nine published articles listed in table 1 are described narratively and their results summarized first according to type of behavioral outcome and then by type of medication used.

Focus on Behavior

The behavioral measures that have been used to study the effects of obstetric medication can generally be divided into ten areas of behavioral functioning (see table 1). These ten areas include the seven conceptual clusters as described by Lester, Als, and Brazelton (1982) (motor, habituation, orientation, reflex, autonomic regulation, range of state, and regulation of state) as well as feeding behavior, social interaction behavior, and electroencephalographic patterns (EEGs).

In considering the results reported here, it should be noted that there are four published articles that have tested separately for statistically significant effects of more than one type of obstetric medication. The results of these studies are tabulated as separate comparisons even though they are reported in one published article. For example reference 23 on table 1 is tabulated as two comparisons: one examining the effects of general anesthesia on infant behavior and one examining the effects of preanesthetic medication on infant behavior. For this reason, the figure given in the text for total number of comparisons finding or failing to find adverse effects sometimes exceeds the actual number of reference numbers that follow that figure.

Motor behavior refers to measures of the infant's integrated motor acts and overall muscle tone. The most frequently used

measures have been motor maturity, defensive movements
(e.g., the infant's attempts to remove a cloth from its upper
face), activity level, amount of head control, arm recoil, and
truncal and general tone.

Motor behavior as a function of maternal obstetric medication has been investigated in thirty-nine comparisons in thirty-
four published studies. Decreased motor performance was reported in twenty-one comparisons (54 percent) (table 1, refs.
5, 8, 12, 17, 18, 23, 24, 25, 26, 27, 29, 36, 37, 40, 43, 47, 48,
51, 54, 56). The remaining eighteen comparisons (46 percent)
(table 1, refs. 1, 2, 3, 4, 6, 15, 23, 28, 34, 38, 41, 42, 49, 53, 56,
58) found that infant motor behavior was not affected by maternal obstetric medication. None of the comparisons reported
enhancement of motor performance.

Habituation is an index of the infant's efficiency of information processing. The infant is exposed to repeated presentation
of a nonmeaningful stimulus (auditory, visual, and tactile stimuli are used most frequently) in order to elicit the orienting
reflex. The examiner records how long it takes the infant to
decrease the rate at which it responds to the redundant stimulation. Most often used measures of orienting and habituation
are respiration, heart rate response, ongoing physical activity,
and turning toward the source of stimulation.

Habituation has been used frequently as a dependent variable in studies of obstetric medication and infant behavior.
There are thirty-nine comparisons in the thirty-three studies in
which it has been included. Maternal obstetric medication was
found to slow habituation in nineteen comparisons (49 percent) (table 1, refs. 2, 8, 9, 12, 17, 18, 22, 23, 24, 25, 26, 27,
39, 41, 48, 55, 56, 59). One of the studies (table 1, ref. 10)
reported a trend toward an impaired habituation response. In
the remaining nineteen comparisons (49 percent) (table 1,
refs. 1, 3, 4, 5, 6, 15, 23, 29, 34, 36, 37, 43, 49, 53, 54, 56, 58),
habituation was not significantly affected by medication. No
comparison found that obstetric medication had a beneficial
effect on infant performance.

The *orienting reflex* is a measure of the infant's initial reaction or responsiveness to a presented stimulus, usually visual or auditory. Orientation is frequently indexed as a change in respiration, heart rate, and ongoing physical activity as well as turning of the eyes and head toward the source of stimulation.

There are forty comparisons in the thirty-seven studies in which orientation has been used to assess the effects of drugs on the infant. Twenty-one of these comparisons (52 percent) (table 1, refs. 5, 6, 8, 12, 14, 17, 23, 24, 25, 26, 27, 29, 37, 40, 43, 47, 52) have reported deficits in orientation as a result of maternal medication. Obstetric medication did not affect orientation in the remaining nineteen comparisons (48 percent) (table 1, refs. 1, 2, 3, 4, 15, 18, 22, 34, 36, 38, 39, 41, 42, 48, 49, 51, 53, 54, 57, 58). There were no findings of improved orienting response in any of the forty comparisons.

The term *reflex behavior* includes measures of elicited responses. Rooting, sucking, Moro, and placing reflexes are reported most frequently in the literature on infant behavior and obstetric medication.

Infant reflex performance following obstetric drug administration has been examined in thirty comparisons in twenty-six studies. Adverse effects on reflex performance due to medication were found in twelve of these comparisons (40 percent) (table 1, refs. 8, 18, 23, 24, 25, 26, 27, 28, 37, 48, 56). Reflex scores were not affected by obstetric medication in the remaining eighteen comparisons (60 percent) (table 1, refs. 1, 2, 3, 4, 6, 15, 23, 36, 38, 41, 42, 43, 49, 53, 54, 56, 58). No comparison found that obstetric medication improved reflex behavior.

Autonomic regulation refers to signs of physiological stress, operationally defined as the number of tremors, startles, and changes in skin color that may take place during a standardized examination.

There are nine comparisons in nine studies in which autonomic regulation has been included as a dependent measure of obstetric medication effects. Impaired performance on autonomic regulation items due to obstetric medication was reported in five comparisons (56 percent) (table 1, refs. 8, 12, 40, 47, 51). Autonomic regulation was not affected by medication in the remaining four (44 percent) (table 1, refs. 2, 15, 29, 54). None of the comparisons reported improved autonomic regulatory function as a result of obstetric medication.

Range of state describes the infant's state pattern (i.e., sleep, awake, alert, crying, quiet, agitated). It is assessed most frequently by observing the infant's predominant states, number of state changes, state control in the presence of aversive stimuli, and irritability during an examination period.

There are seventeen comparisons in sixteen studies examining the effects of obstetric medication on range of state. Of these, ten comparisons (59 percent) (table 1, refs. 5, 8, 12, 21, 29, 46, 47, 51, 57, 59) found significant, detrimental change in range of state following obstetric medication whereas seven comparisons (41 percent) (table 1, refs. 1, 2, 15, 34, 54, 55) found that obstetric medication had no effect on range of state. None of the seventeen comparisons reported that maternal drug administration improved performance on items used to assess range of state.

Lester et al. (1982) refer to *regulation of state* as the infant's ability to modulate his or her states of consciousness. It is assessed most often by items from Brazelton's (1973) Neonatal Behavioral Assessment Scale (e.g., self-quieting activity, consolability with intervention).

The effect of obstetric medication on state regulation has been examined in eleven comparisons in ten studies. Decreased abilities to modulate state were found in seven of these comparisons (64 percent) (table 1, refs. 5, 8, 29, 40, 47, 54, 57) and nonsignificant effects in four comparisons (36 percent) (table 1, refs. 2, 12, 34). No comparison found that obstetric medication increased the infant's ability to regulate its own state.

Feeding behavior has been used to measure the effects of obstetric medication in twenty-eight comparisons in twenty-three studies. Frequently used measures of feeding behavior include strength of rooting and sucking reflexes, sucking rate and pressure, number and length of feeding intervals, amount consumed, and responsiveness to feeding. Obstetric medication was followed by significant, detrimental effects on feeding behavior in seventeen of these comparisons (61 percent) (table 1, refs. 11, 20, 23, 24, 25, 26, 27, 28, 32, 33, 37, 40, 45, 48, 56) but not in the remaining eleven (39 percent) (table 1, refs. 1, 3, 4, 14, 18, 49, 53, 54, 56, 59). No investigation has found feeding behavior to be enhanced by drug administration.

Social interaction has generally been measured by observing parent and infant behavior during feeding and nonfeeding periods. The behaviors most commonly used to assess social interaction are the frequency and amount of time the parents spend talking to, looking at, smiling at, touching, holding, kissing, rocking, and establishing eye contact with their infants as well as the infant's responsiveness to these behaviors.

There are eight comparisons in seven studies that have examined the influence of obstetric medication on social interaction. Obstetric medication disrupted interaction in five, or 62 percent of these comparisons (table 1, refs. 5, 11, 34, 40, 45), but had no significant effect in the other three comparisons (38 percent) (table 1, refs. 14, 34, 44). Obstetric medication has never been found to improve or increase social interaction.

Electroencephalography (EEG) measures the electrical activity of the brain. Infant EEG patterns have been used as a dependent measure of obstetric medication effects in four comparisons in four studies. All four, or 100 percent, of these comparisons (table 1, refs. 7, 13, 30, 31) found that obstetric medication significantly changed patterns of brain wave activity. In the study by Brower et al. (table 1, ref. 13) EEG changes were found during presentation of auditory stimulation. However, spontaneous brain activity and evoked response to visual, tactile, and olfactory stimuli were not significantly affected.

Focus on Drugs

The obstetric drugs that have been used in the fifty-nine studies summarized in table 1 are generally classified as pre-anesthetic, local anesthetic, and general anesthetic medications. Table 1 also includes a designation of "mixed" for comparisons examining the effects of any combination of these three on infant behavior. Generally speaking, the intended use of these medications is to control pain during labor and delivery. Examples of each group are given below in the report of results according to type of drug.

In considering the results reported below, it should be noted that the majority of the fifty-nine published articles examine the effects of obstetric medication on more than one type of behavior. The effect of a particular type of medication on each of the behavioral variables examined in a published article is tabulated as a separate comparison of that drug's effect on infant behavior. For example, Belsey et al. (table 1, ref. 5) is tabulated as six separate comparisons of the effects of preanesthetic medication on infant behavior, i.e., the effect of preanesthetic medication on motor, habituation, orientation, range of state, regulation of state, and social interaction behaviors. Since most published articles include more than one measure of behavior, the figure given in the text for the total number of comparisons that found or failed to find adverse effects exceeds the actual number of referenced studies following that figure. As a final note, those comparisons examining the effects of *mixed medication* (some combination of preanesthetic, local anesthetic, and general anesthetic medication) were not included in the tabulation of results for outcome by type of drug since the effects, or lack of effects, on infant behavior could not be attributed to any one of the three types of obstetric medication.

The effects of *preanesthetic medication* on infant behavior have been examined in eighty-two comparisons in twenty-three studies. The most frequently studied preanesthetic medications have been narcotic analgesics (e.g., meperidine, morphine); sedative-hypnotics including both the barbiturates (e.g., pentobarbital, phenobarbital, secobarbital) and the nonbarbiturates (e.g., diazepam, scopolamine); and tranquilizers (e.g., the phenothiazine derivatives: promethazine, promazine, chloropromazine). Of the eighty-two comparisons examining the effect of preanesthetic medication on infant behavior, fifty-one (table 1, refs. 5, 6, 7, 8, 9, 11, 13, 14, 16, 18, 23, 25, 27, 30, 31, 33, 45, 52, 56, 57), or 62 percent, found that preanesthetic medication impaired the behavior tested. Of the eighty-two comparisons, thirty-one, or 38 percent (table 1, refs. 5, 6, 14, 15, 18, 23, 34, 56, 57, 58), found that preanesthetic medication did not affect the behavior tested. None of the eighty-two comparisons found that infant behavior was improved by preanesthetic medication.

The effect of *local anesthesia* on infant behavior has been assessed in sixty comparisons in fifteen studies. The most frequently studied local anesthetics include bupivacaine, lidocaine, mepivacaine, and tetracaine (amide compounds) and procaine and chloroprocaine (ester compounds). Twenty-seven comparisons or 45 percent (table 1, refs. 28, 34, 36, 37, 40, 41, 46, 47, 48, 56) found that local anesthesia lowered performance on one or more of the behaviors tested. In the remaining thirty-three comparisons (55 percent) (table 1, refs. 1, 19, 28, 34, 35, 36, 37, 38, 41, 48, 49, 56) local anesthesia did not affect the behavior studied. Local anesthetics did not improve behavioral performance in any of the sixty comparisons.

The effect of *general anesthetics* on infant behavior has been examined in twenty-seven comparisons in six studies. Those general anesthetics used most frequently were nitrous oxide, methoxyflurane, thiopental, and ketamine. Of these twenty-seven, twenty-five comparisons, or 93 percent (table 1, refs. 23, 24, 26, 27, 39), found that general anesthesia impaired performance on one or more of the behaviors tested. Two comparisons, or 7 percent (table 1, refs. 39, 50), found that general anesthesia did not affect infant behavior. None of the comparisons found that behavioral performance was enhanced by general anesthesia.

Summary and Conclusions

The results of the studies listed in table 1 may be summarized as follows.

- Drugs administered to mothers during labor and delivery significantly affect infant behavior. Of the fifty-nine published articles listed in table 1, forty-seven found that obstetric medication significantly affected one or more infant behaviors.
- All the studies finding significant effects of obstetric medication on infant behavior have found these effects to be detrimental. No study found that obstetric medication enhanced or improved infant behavior.
- For eight of the ten areas of behavior, more than half the comparisons showed that significant, adverse behavioral effects followed the administration of obstetric medication.
- There is more evidence for obstetric medication effects in some areas of behavioral functioning than in others. The areas of behavioral functioning (and the percentage of the comparisons that found significant drug effects on that area of behavioral functioning) follow in rank order, from highest to lowest: EEG (100 percent), regulation of state (64 percent), social interaction (62 percent), feeding (61 percent), range of state (59 percent), autonomic regulation (56 percent), motor behavior (54 percent), orientation (52 percent), habituation (49 percent), and reflex behavior (40 percent).
- There is evidence that the potency or total burden of the obstetric drug administered is related to the extent of behavioral effects. General anesthesia, the most potent of the three types of obstetric medication, adversely affected

behavior in twenty-five of the twenty-seven comparisons (93 percent) in which its effects were tested. Preanesthetic agents, also distributed systemically but less potent than general anesthetic agents, were linked to impaired behavior in fifty-one of eighty-two comparisons (62 percent). Local anesthesia had the least impact on behavior: only twenty-seven of the sixty comparisons (45 percent) found significant effects of these agents on infant behavior.

In evaluating the seriousness of the problem of obstetric medication, it is important to bear in mind that the impairments produced by behavioral teratogens are characteristically subtle ones, difficult to identify and to measure reliably, particularly in infants. Nonsignificant findings do not necessarily mean that the behavior in question was unaffected. If there existed more sensitive and reliable measures of infant behavior and inferential statistics more suitable for detecting low-level effects, it is likely that significant findings would increase substantially.

It is also important to remember that the behavioral problems caused by obstetric medication may extend well beyond the early period of development. As noted earlier, few studies of obstetric medication and infant behavior have tested for effects beyond six weeks of age, and no studies have tested beyond the first year. The general problems associated with a longitudinal design (e.g., amount of time and money required; subject attrition), as well as a lack of age-equivalent measures, have resulted in a noticeable absence of studies of long-term effects following early exposure to obstetric medication.

Nevertheless, a lack of studies does not mean a lack of lasting effects. When early damage occurs, it may be compensated to some extent. However, the damage-compensated organism usually does not perform as well as the nondamaged organism under all environmental conditions. Ucko (1965) found that children who had suffered perinatal anoxia functioned as well as normal children in everyday situations but

xhibited more behavioral disturbances in stressful situations.
The limitations of compensatory mechanisms under demand-
ng conditions have also been demonstrated in the animal lit-
rature. Simons, Puretz, and Finger (1975) and Finger and
Simons (1976) found that sequentially brain-lesioned rats per-
ormed as well as normal controls on an easy tactile discrimination task but more poorly than normals when task difficulty
vas increased.

Although there are no long-term studies in the human literature, there are reports in the animal literature of permanent
deficits resulting from early exposure to drugs. For example,
seroff (1980) briefly exposed infant rats to hydroxyzine (a tran-
quilizer frequently administered during childbirth) and found
that it impaired their ability to learn as adults.

In many of the studies of obstetric medication and human
infant behavior reviewed above, deficits in efficiency of information processing (habituation) and attention (orienting reflex) were found. The significance and implications of these
findings become even greater when one considers the strong
probability of permanent effects. Dysfunction in the neurophysiological processes mediating these infant behaviors may be
reflected later in development as deficits in more complex behaviors, including disorders of learning.

CHAPTER 2

Medical Decision Making: Information as Power

A Short History of Medical Disclosure

Withholding information from patients has a long history in the medical profession. The same physician who gave medicine its ethic also enjoined his colleagues to "conceal most things from the patient. . . .reveal nothing of the patient's future or present condition." Providing information, according to Hippocrates, caused many patients to "take a turn for the worse" (Pernick 1982, 4). Such a view, nurtured through the ages, finally blossomed into what is now known as "medical paternalism." As one medical historian put it, by the early nineteenth century "the majority of practitioners appear to have regarded liberty as more likely to be pathogenic than therapeutic" (Pernick 1982, 7). Speaking for this majority, Thouvenel wrote

> It is important for the happiness of all that man be placed under the sacred power of the physician. That he be brought up, nourished, clothed after his counsel and that the systems according to which he should be governed, educated, punished, etc., be designed by him. . . . Who is better qualified to play this role than the physician who has made a profound study of his physical and moral nature? (Pernick 1982, 7)

Yet, even if they constituted a minority of physicians, there were those who held, as early as the late eighteenth century, that individual health was directly promoted by individual liberty, including informed decision making. In the United States, a leading proponent of disclosure was Benjamin Rush, who advised his fellow physicians to "strip our profession of everything that looks like mystery and imposture, and clothe medical knowledge in a dress so simple and intelligible, that it may become . . . obvious to the meanest capacities" (Pernick 1982, 6).

Despite the predominant view favoring nondisclosure, most early physicians found it necessary in practice to inform their conscious patients about their conditions and to obtain their consents to treatment. The need to do so, however, decreased with the advent of specialized medical knowledge and technologies, particularly drugs and other agents that temporarily interfere with consciousness and mental competence. This was exemplified by the discovery of anesthesia in the mid-nineteenth century—a discovery that widened the power gap between physician and patient in one great quantum leap. Textbooks of the times instructed that anesthesia's "benefits are not confined to the abolition of pain:. . . it circumvents the opposition of the timid and unruly" (Pernick 1982, 22). Among those regularly regarded by nineteenth-century physicians as timid, unruly, or otherwise incompetent to decide upon their own course of treatment were slaves, immigrants, and women. Obstetricians found ether and chloroform the perfect accessory in deflecting any resistance their female patients might dare to show, as the following quotation from 1862 illustrates.

Now, sir, in forceps cases, . . . Chloroform is of great advantage in enabling you to make a thorough examination of the child without the mother's knowing that you are doing so. . . . Another advantage consists in the fact that you can have a consultation without her knowing it. . . . the [consulting] doctor can come, perform the operation and retire, while the patient is utterly ignorant of what is being done. (Pernick 1982, 23)

Currently, though doctors may be more guarded in their statements about disclosure and shared decision making, it is clear from a recent Harris poll (Harris, Boyle, and Brounstein 1982), carried out at the request of the President's Commission, that medical paternalism still predominates over informed consent. In this study, the majority (56 percent) of physicians surveyed felt that they were justified in withholding information from some patients. A majority (54 percent) also reported that they find themselves at least once a day deliberating how much to tell a patient about his or her condition. A very large majority (88 percent) stated a belief that their patients want them to choose the treatment alternative. Akin to their attitudes about informed consent was physicians' knowledge of informed consent. In answer to the question "What does the term 'informed consent' mean to you?" only 59 percent responded that it involved giving patients information about their conditions and possible treatments, and only 9 percent stated that informed consent bore on patients making decisions or indicating their preference among treatment alternatives.

Informed Consent: Moral Duty, Legal Mandate

The right to participate in decisions affecting one's own well-being and the right to have information relevant to those decisions are two inextricably bound rights that have been transformed from age-old ethical values to a recently defined legal doctrine called *informed consent.* Informed consent requires health care practitioners to provide patients with all information on proposed treatments or procedures bearing on the decision to accept or reject treatments.[5] Such information includes the nature and purpose of the procedure, its probable

---

5. In terms of denotative precision, *informed decision* would be a more appropriate term than *informed consent.* The latter term was used originally in recruiting subjects for research.

benefits, its possible risks (including side effects), and treatment alternatives, including their benefits and risks. Additional elements of the informed consent doctrine are that the decision (consent or refusal) must be voluntary; that the patient must be competent to decide; that the patient must understand the information presented; that the decision must be made by the patient; and that the health care provider must respect that decision (Lidz and Roth 1983).

Only the term and legal doctrine of informed consent are new. The underlying rights themselves have a history as long as the existence of societies respecting personal freedom and as long as the existence of ethicists within those societies. From the categorical imperatives of Immanuel Kant came the deontological position. From the perspective of deontology, informed consent is justified because it promotes the person's autonomy or self-determination.[6] The other major ethical tradition, utilitarianism, holds that the consequences of an act determine its morality. To be morally right, the benefits of an act must exceed its costs. Thus, from the utilitarian point of view, informed consent is justified by the fact that it promotes the person's well-being.

These two values, respect for autonomy and respect for well-being, are the ethical positions. How well are ethics sustained in fact? In the sections that follow, we examine the empirical documentation concerning the use of informed consent in medicine in general and obstetrics in particular.

Respect for Autonomy: The Right to Be Informed

The first of three empirical studies (Lidz and Meisel 1982) authorized by the President's Commission on Ethical Problems in Medicine had as its purpose to determine whether and how

---

6. A second justification for informed consent, from the deontological perspective, stems from the fact that it promotes another value basic to the successful functioning of free societies, namely *rationality:* Providing information facilitates the person's coming to a rational decision.

decision making and communication actually take place between patients and health care professionals under a variety of real-life medical circumstances.

The investigators anticipated that, in accordance with the legal model of informed consent, information would be *disclosed* to patients; that patients would *understand* that information; that patients would *decide* to undergo (consent) or forego (refuse) the procedure in question; and that patients would act *voluntarily* in making that decision. Instead, they found something quite different. They found that medical personnel do not see patient participation or the handling of consent forms as part of the decision-making process but rather as a legal formality and bureaucratic nuisance. Consent forms are preprinted, with general, all-inclusive, legally oriented wording. Further, they are always presented to patients after the treatment decision has already been made and usually just before that treatment is about to take place. In fact, informed consent is not even sought for "routine" treatments (including drug administration), and it is just such routine treatment that characterizes almost all aspects of traditional, in-hospital delivery.

Lidz and Meisel conclude that "the manner in which decisions are made . . . bears little resemblance to the decision making process contemplated by the informed consent doctrine" (1982, 340). They go on to point out, "This stands the traditional doctrine of informed consent on its head" (p. 400). Instead of the ethical/legal presumption that the patient will not be touched unless s(he) has given permission, doctors presume that they are free to initiate their procedures unless the patient objects. "Consent," as the investigators point out, "does not exist." Instead, what we find is "acquiescence" and "the absence of 'objection' " (p. 401).

A second investigation (Appelbaum and Roth 1982) authorized by the President's Commission on Ethical Problems in Medicine was an observational study of treatment refusals in medical hospital wards, including a gynecological unit. The investigators found that the major precipitating factors in normal adult patients' refusing treatment was that medical personnel had failed to inform them about the purpose or risk of a treatment or had failed to inform them that the treatment had been ordered at all. After information was provided, most patients withdrew their refusals and consented to treatment. Both outcomes led to the conclusion that disclosure increases rather than decreases compliance.

Another major reason for treatment refusals stemmed from conflicting information given patients. As the commissioners noted, this is particularly likely to happen in hospitals "where patient care is divided among different people, many of whom are not in direct communication with each other" (President's Commission 1982, 80).

A third study (Harris, Boyle, and Brounstein 1982) done for the President's Commission on Ethical Problems in Medicine conducted parallel national surveys of 805 physicians and 1,251 adults concerning their knowledge, attitudes, and experiences relating to disclosure and decision making in therapeutic settings. Harris and his associates found large and consistent differences between the proportion of doctors reporting disclosure to patients on various aspects of their medical care and the proportion of patients reporting that their doctors provide that information. For example, 93 percent of the doctors surveyed reported that they usually discuss those side effects, including inconvenience and pain, that are certain or fairly certain to result from a particular treatment, whereas only 68 percent of the public report that their doctors usually discuss such side effects.

As another illustration, although 94 percent of the public wants to be told everything about their condition and treatment, even if the news is unfavorable, 56 percent of doctors believe that some patients should be told less than other patients and that they themselves should decide which patients should be provided with how much information. Only 17 percent of the physicians polled believe that all their patients wanted full information about their diagnoses and prognoses (President's Commission 1982, 75).

The only agreement between doctors and patients on the extent to which physicians provide information was the economic issue of costs and insurance coverage: 47 percent of doctors reported that they usually discussed this with their patients; 45 percent of the patient respondents agreed.

Harris and associates also queried doctors on their knowledge of the legal standards for informed consent applicable to the state in which they practiced. A large majority (76 percent) of these physicians freely admitted they were not familiar with their state's standards, and a substantial number (32 percent) of those who thought they knew the applicable standard did not.

Respect for Well-Being

From the utilitarian perspective, the main justification for informed consent is the fact that it promotes the individual's well-being. Informed consent is morally right because its benefits exceed its costs.

Such a position lends itself to empirical test. From the health research evidence available, what support is there to show that the informed decision maker is better off than the individual who is deprived of information and decision-making opportunities?

Informed Decision Making: Rx for Health

Numerous studies have examined the effects of providing health consumers with information important to their welfare and with the opportunity to use that information in a decision-making capacity. Studies focusing on physiological responses to the provision of information have found, for example, that informed patients respond to medical procedures with less distress than their uninformed counterparts (Mills and Krantz

1979; Saunderson 1977), report less pain (Putt 1970), need fewer narcotics and other drugs (Egbert et al. 1964; Seltzer, Roncari, and Garfinkel 1980), are more apt to change from a hypertensive to a normotensive state (McKenney et al. 1973), and show improved courses of recovery, including shorter periods of hospitalization (Egbert et al. 1964; Janis 1958; Putt 1970).

Other studies in this area have focused on the effects of information or informed consent on compliance. The impetus for such studies has been physicians' widely expressed belief that disclosing negative information leads to noncompliance and their widely held practice of withholding information on these grounds. In these investigations, compliance is operationally defined as accepting and adhering to treatment recommendations (particularly, consuming prescribed drugs). By far the majority of studies have found that providing information increases compliance (Colcher and Bass 1972; Gotsch and Liguori 1982; Korsch and Negrete 1972; MacDonald, MacDonald, and Phoenix 1977; McKenney et al. 1973; Norell 1979; Seltzer, Roncari, and Garfinkel 1980; Sharpe and Mikeal 1974; Svarsted 1976). A few studies have found that information has no significant effect on compliance (e.g., Myers and Calvert 1973, 1976). Medical convictions to the contrary, no study has found that providing information and decision-making opportunities reduces compliance.

Another consistent finding from investigations in this area is that providing information and some degree of control through decision making increases patients' satisfaction with their health care (Bertakis 1977; Comstock et al. 1982; Gillette, Byrne, and Cranton 1982; Korsch and Negrete 1972; Ley et al. 1976).

Several investigations have examined the effects of providing patients with information concerning possible side effects of their medication. These studies have consistently found that informed patients are no more apt to report side effects than uninformed patients (Morris and Kanouse 1982; Myers and

Calvert 1973, 1976; Paulson et al. 1976). MacDonald, MacDonald, and Phoenix (1977) found the providing information greatly reduced self-generated medication errors among the elderly.

In a remarkable series of experimental studies of the institutionalized elderly, investigators have found that experimental subjects given even small increments of decision-making control and responsibility for their own lives become happier, more active, more alert, and more sociable than subjects not given control (Langer and Rodin 1976; Pohl and Fuller 1980). They also show a decreased need for medication (Schulz 1976), improved general health (Rodin and Langer 1977; Schulz 1976), and lower mortality rates (Rodin and Langer 1977). (For a review of the research, see Rodin, Bohm, and Wack 1982.)

Just as research consistently indicates that providing information and decision-making opportunities has positive consequences for mental and physical health, so does it also consistently show that depriving people of information and the power to make decisions in matters bearing on their own welfare is associated with a variety of adverse psychological and physiological consequences. Within the first category, loss of control and information has been shown to produce such negative emotional responses as anger, anxiety, apathy, depression, extreme passivity, or "learned helplessness" (Friedman, Greenspan, and Mittleman 1974; Seligman 1975) and generalized feelings of dehumanization and demoralization (Price 1977; Shaw 1974). Negative consequences on cognitive functioning include decreased learning and coping abilities (Seligman 1975) and decreased ability to process new information efficiently, objectively, and validly (Janis and Mann 1977). Adverse motivational effects found to be associated with informational deficit and loss of decision-making control are especially apt to lead to noncompliance (Appelbaum and Roth 1982; Boyd et al. 1974; Fitzpatrick and Hopkins 1981; Janis 1958; Korsch and Negrete 1972), to nondiscriminating demands for health-related information (see review by Taylor 1979), and to dissatisfaction with health care (Janis 1958; Kirke 1980).

Physiological consequences stemming from withholding information and decision-making opportunities include signs of stress, including elevated catecholamine excretion followed by adrenaline depletion (Seligman 1975) and increased mortality among the elderly (Rodin and Langer 1977).

The studies noted above on the consequences of providing or withholding information and decision-making control are studies of human beings in real-life, health care settings. For reviews of laboratory studies that have investigated the same topics and that have used college students or animals as subjects, the reader is referred to Garber and Seligman 1980, and Wortman and Brehm 1975.

CHAPTER 3

The Florida Study

In this study we investigated maternal drug consumption and infant drug exposure during pregnancy and childbirth, the status of those drugs with respect to adverse fetal effects, and the amount of information mothers have about the drugs they have consumed.

Participants

Participants were 602 postpartum women: 402 women who chose traditional, in-hospital delivery under the care of an obstetrician; 100 women who chose out-of-hospital delivery at a birth center with the aid of a nurse midwife; and 100 who chose to deliver at home with the aid of an empirical midwife.

The traditionally delivered mothers, henceforth referred to as *Hospital Mothers,* were obstetric inpatients at the University of Florida's Shands Teaching Hospital, Gainesville. These women were randomly chosen from all obstetric patients available on any interview day who had borne babies classified by the obstetrical staff as clinically normal and as having Apgar scores of at least 3 at one minute and 5 at five minutes postpartum.[7] Since the obstetrical unit encourages low-risk, vaginally delivered mothers to leave as soon as possible after delivery, the final sample contained a disproportionately high number of surgically delivered mothers—35 percent, which is 15 percent higher than the hospital's actual cesarean section rate. The average prenatal risk

---

7. The Apgar score is a system of evaluation that describes the status of the infant at one and five minutes after birth with respect to heart rate, breathing effort, muscle tone, reflex irritability, and color.

score for vaginally delivered mothers was .36 and that for surgically delivered mothers, .62. Other demographic characteristics of Hospital Mothers, as well as those birthing out-of-hospital, are shown in chapter 4 (see table 2).

All mothers who participated in this research project gave their written, informed consent prior to being interviewed. The content and format of the consent had been approved by the university's J. H. Miller Health Center Committee for the Protection of Human Subjects. Each mother received a duplicate copy of the written consent form.

A brief, postinterview evaluation was carried out with 106 of the 402 Hospital Mothers a few hours after the interview had been completed. The evaluation was carried out by student volunteers who were not members of the research team and who were naive with respect to the purpose of the research other than that it dealt with "medications." Each mother was asked whether she had liked or disliked the interview as a whole or in part, whether there was anything disturbing about the interview, and how she felt it would be received by other mothers in the obstetric unit.

A second group of 100 mothers, referred to as *Center Mothers,* chose to deliver at a freestanding birth center in Gainesville or Daytona, Florida.

Freestanding birth center programs offer complete prenatal, birthing, and postpartum care. Their programs emphasize the active participation of women and their partners in the childbirth process. Birth takes place in a comfortably furnished, homelike bedroom and may be attended by siblings, other family members, and friends.

Clients are carefully screened for acceptance into a birth center program. Centers generally accept only those who are "low risk," defined in terms of medical history, current health, and motivation. Center staff continue to monitor risk status throughout pregnancy and delivery, referring those clients who develop risk problems at any stage to the hospital for traditional care.

Although birth centers employ physicians on an ad hoc cor sulting basis, certified nurse midwives are the primary pro viders of health care. Certified nurse midwives are registere nurses who have had one to two years of training in a nurs midwifery program and who have been certified by the Amer can College of Nurse Midwives.

At the time the present study was being conducted, th charge for prenatal care, delivery, and postnatal care was on thousand dollars at both the Gainesville and Daytona center:

The names of Center Mothers were obtained from birt certificates filed with the State Records Office. Of the 1C mothers contacted, 2 declined to participate. Mothers wer interviewed in their own homes after obtaining informe consent. All babies born to Center Mother participants ha been classified by the nurse midwife attendant as clinical normal.

The third group of mothers, referred to as *Home Mothe* had chosen to deliver at home with the assistance of an empi: cal midwife (sometimes called a "lay" midwife). Empiric midwives represent 90 to 95 percent of all midwives in Floric according to Florida Midwives Association statistics.[8] Th training consists of self-instruction and an apprenticeship two to three years with an experienced empirical midwife. Fe have working relationships with physicians. According to t association, the average empirical midwife in Florida is thin years old and has been practicing for five years. Most empi cal midwives offer total care, i.e., prenatal care, childbin education, delivery, and postnatal care, for an average fee five hundred dollars. This fee is not currently reimbursed health insurance companies.

As with Center Mothers, the names of mothers delivering home were obtained from State Records Office birth cert cates. Of the 102 potential participating Home Mothers

8. Linda Wilson, President, Florida Midwives Association, personal c munication, September, 1982.

declined to be interviewed. Mothers were intereviewed in their own homes after obtaining informed consent. All babies born to Home Mothers had been classed as clinically normal by the attending midwife.

Sources of Data

The principal source of data was a structured interview which focused on health-related problems experienced during pregnancy; the ways, including drug therapy, in which participants coped with those problems; amount and source of information about drugs consumed prenatally; drug administration during labor and delivery; amount of information about obstetric drugs; information about drugs in general; engagement in health-promoting behaviors; and demographic variables. Another data source was the Rotter Locus of Control Scale (Rotter 1966).

Health-Related Complaints during Pregnancy: Drug Exposure and Information

The mother was first asked about any health-related problems she might have experienced during pregnancy (see chap. 4, table 3). If she reported that a problem had occurred, the interviewer asked whether it had been treated. If it had not been treated, the interviewer asked why. If it had been treated, the interviewer asked how. When a mother reported that she had used a medication to treat a problem, she was asked what information she had about the medication and where she had gotten that information.

Guidelines used in probing for information as well as scoring for amount and accuracy of that information were those endorsed by the American Society of Hospital Pharmacists (1976) as basic points of information that consumers should know about every drug they consume (see chap. 4, table 18). In other words, for each drug reportedly consumed, mothers were asked to specify its name, intended use, directions for administration, special directions for preparation, precautions to be observed, common side effects, techniques for self-monitoring, therapeutic contraindications including interactions, and miscellaneous information including refill and missed dose information, etc. These points of consumer information are basically the same as those recommended for patient information to the U.S. Pharmacopoeia by their conference of delegates in 1970 and as incorporated into the newly published *United States Pharmacopoeia Dispensing Information for Patients* (1980).

In tabulating mothers' responses, correct information was scored positively; incorrect, negatively. Scores ranged from a possible +9 to −9. To adjust for differing numbers of pregnancy-related complaints and thus differing numbers of occasions for drug therapy, a mean information score was obtained by averaging across all drugs consumed during pregnancy.

Mothers were also asked about the source of information for each drug consumed during pregnancy, i.e., whether she had gotten the information from a friend or relative; a magazine or newspaper; a package label; a pharmacist; a physician; a television program or commercial; or from some other source. Specific inquiry was also made about books and articles, childbirth education classes, and physicians as general sources of information, and about desire for information about drugs to be consumed.

Drug Exposure and Information during Labor
and Delivery

The interviewer next asked the mother about any medications she might have received during labor and delivery. For each medication reported, the mother was asked if she knew what it was, how it had been given, and what information she had about it. Her account of medication administration was compared to the medical records account.

Information about Drugs in General

This measure, incorporated into the interview as a subset of
twelve items, assessed mothers' knowledge about a standard
set of drugs, thus allowing comparison across respondents
regardless of individual differences in medical conditions that
may have required medication. The twelve items included
six substances commonly used outside obstetrics and known
to be or suspected of being teratogenic (amphetamine, aspirin, caffeine, Darvon [propoxyphene], diethylstilbestrol
[DES], and Dilantin [phenytoin]) and six drugs frequently
administered during childbirth (Doering and Stewart 1978)
(Demerol [meperidine], Xylocaine [lidocaine], Nisentil [al-
phaprodine], nitrous oxide, Phenergan [promethazine], and
Vistaril [hydroxyzine]).

Instructions were, "We're interested in finding out how
much information people have about medications. Here are
the points of information we're interested in. Here is a list of
medications. Please tell me everything you know about each of
them." Responses were scored using a relevant subset of the
nine points of information used in scoring information about
drugs actually consumed.

Health-Promoting Behaviors

Interspersed among the other interview questions were
twenty-four items collectively termed *health-promoting behaviors*. Adapted from a set developed by the Canadian Minis-
try of Health, these items assess the extent to which the
respondent behaves in ways known to promote health and
prevent illness or disease, and over which she has control,
e.g., avoidance of smoking and alcohol consumption, maintenance of appropriate weight for height, use of seat belts,
breast self-examination, etc.

The entire set of health-promoting behaviors is shown in

Appendix A. The theoretical range of scores for this measure was 96 points, with high scores indicating more participation in health-promoting practices.

Demographic Variables

The interview concluded by gathering relevant background information, including age, number of children borne by interviewee, education, religious affiliation, living arrangement, and receipt of financial assistance.

Locus of Control

Following the interview, if time permitted, the Rotter Locus of Control Scale (Rotter 1966) was administered. This scale was devised to measure the extent to which respondents perceive life events to be under their own control ("internal" locus of control) as opposed to the extent to which they perceive life events as being the consequence of social constraints, vagaries of fate, or actions of others ("external" locus of control). Scores range from 0 (maximum internal control) to 23 (maximum external control).

Inclusion of this scale was prompted by the results of many studies showing that perceived locus of control predicts informational parameters of the sort under investigation in the present research. Specifically, research in this area has found that subjects with highly internal scores also show higher information scores; greater willingness to be exposed to information, independent of ability; and more effective and efficient use of information (Lefcourt 1976; Lefcourt and Wine 1969; Prociuk and Breen 1977; Russo 1977; Russo, Krieser, and Miyashita 1975; Seeman 1963; Seeman and Evans 1962; Waitzkin and Stoeckle 1976). We therefore hypothesized that locus of control scale scores would predict amount of information about drugs.

Interviewers

There were eight interviewers, all of whom were trained extensively by means of role-playing techniques and supervised practice interviews. Of the eight, seven were women, five were advanced students, and two, midwives. There were no ascertainable differences in quality or quantity of responses as a function of interviewer's sex or occupation. All interviewers were white, whereas approximately 32 percent of the interviewees were black. Published literature indicates that matching interviewer and interviewee by race is advisable only when the interview content concerns race-related issues (Sudman and Bradburn 1974).

Upon its completion, each interview was coded by the interviewer. It was then coded independently by a senior member of the research team who resolved any coding disagreements with the interviewer.

CHAPTER 4

The Evidence

Demographic Characteristics

Demographic data for the three groups of mothers are shown in table 2. These measures are considered outcome variables since all mothers available within the time constraints of the study were included as participants.

As the figures in table 2 indicate, there were significant overall differences among groups on each demographic measure except one, that of the number of self-reported, health-related problems during pregnancy.

With respect to age and parity, Center Mothers were, on the average, the oldest of the three groups (though they were not significantly older than Home Mothers). Despite their older age, they had significantly fewer children than did Hospital or Home Mothers. For most Center Mothers, the subject child was their first. More than one-half of the Hospital Mothers and two-thirds of the Home Mothers had already experienced one birth.

In years of education, Center Mothers significantly outranked Home Mothers by nine months [$t(198) = 2.99$, $p < .003$] and Hospital Mothers by 3.3 years [$t(498) = 15.06$, $p < .0001$].

There were striking differences in ethnic origin between Hospital Mothers, on the one hand, and Center and Home Mothers, on the other. In the hospital sample, 52 percent of participants were white; 47 percent black; and 1 percent American Indian. Among Center and Home Mothers, 98 percent and 93 percent of the respective samples were white.

TABLE 2. Demographic Data

Measure	Hospital Mothers ($N = 402$)	Center Mothers ($N = 100$)	Home Mothers ($N = 100$)	Statistical Comparison
Age in years (M)	22.72 (5.48)	27.28 (4.50)	26.57 (4.06)	$F(2,587) = 43.96^{**}$
Parity (N)				$X^2(8) = 19.83^{*}$
One child	185 (46)	58 (58)	29 (29)	
Two children	108 (27)	25 (25)	42 (42)	
Three or more children	109 (27)	17 (17)	29 (29)	
Education in years (M)	11.27 (1.98)	14.58 (1.93)	13.71 (2.70)	$F(2,586) = 142.07^{**}$
Ethnic origin (number of white mothers)	209 (52)	98 (98)	93 (93)	$X^2(2) = 107.34^{**}$
Religion (N)				$X^2(4) = 85.57^{**}$
Traditional[a]	276 (69)	45 (45)	25 (25)	
Nontraditional	57 (14)	21 (21)	50 (50)	
None	69 (17)	34 (34)	25 (25)	
Living arrangements (N)				$X^2(2) = 104.56^{**}$
With baby's father	233 (58)	100 (100)	98 (98)	
Without baby's father	169 (42)		2 (2)	

Worked while pregnant (N)	253 (63)	90 (90)	83 (83)	$X^2(2) = 37.03$**
Full time	167 (42)	70 (70)	55 (55)	$X^2(2) = 155.52$**
Received aid while pregnant	272 (68)	8 (8)	19 (19)	
Pregnant health status				
Complaints (M)	5.43 (2.50)	5.25 (1.78)	4.84 (2.23)	NS
Risks				
Prenatal (M)	0.47 (.73)	0.15 (.44)	0.16 (.47)	
Perinatal (M)	0.53 (.76)	0.10 (.36)	0.07 (.30)	
None (prenatal and perinatal) (N)	160 (40)	83 (83)	82 (82)	$X^2(2) = 72.34$**
Delivery by section	150 (37)	0	0	

Note: Descriptive entries are numbers (N) with percentage given in parentheses or means (M) with standard deviation given in parentheses.

[a]Protestant, Catholic, Jewish
*$p \leq .01$ **$p \leq .0001$

Among the remaining, 3 were American Indians; 2 Oriental; and 4 black.

There were also marked differences among the three groups in religious affiliation. Most of the Hospital Mothers were affiliated with Protestant churches of a traditional mold, principally Baptists. Among Center Mothers, traditional Protestant ties were the most frequently encountered religious affiliations, but next most frequently encountered were no ties at all. The proportion of Center Mothers reporting no religious affiliation was substantially higher than among the other two groups. Choice of religion among Home Mothers was notable for its nontraditional character; exactly half of these participants belonged to such groups as Jehovah's Witnesses, Latter-Day Saints, Pentecostal, Scientologist, or Eastern religions.

With two exceptions, all Center and Home Mothers were living with the baby's father at the time of the interview. In contrast, 42 percent of the Hospital Mothers were single parents. Within the group of single parents, 130 (or 77.1 percent) were black and 39 (or 22.9 percent) white.

Most of the 602 participants worked while pregnant. Employment was lowest and financial aid highest among Hospital Mothers, many of whom received food stamps or were involved in the state-sponsored program called Women and Infant Care (WIC).

Health-Related Problems and Coping Strategies

The number of health-related problems that mothers reported having occurred during their pregnancies did not differ among groups (table 3). However, there were very large differences between Hospital Mothers, on the one hand, and Center and Home Mothers, on the other, in terms of number of prenatal and intrapartal risks reported (in their medical records) by health personnel (tables 4 and 5). No apparent risks were reported in medical records for 64.7 percent of Hospital Mothers, 88.0 percent of Center Mothers, and 87.2 percent of

Home Mothers. The mean number of prenatal risk factors cited were .47 for Hospital Mothers, .15 for Center Mothers, and .16 for Home Mothers.

None of the Center or Home Mothers underwent surgical delivery, but 150, or 37 percent, of the Hospital respondents did so. The mean number of intrapartal risks for Hospital Mothers delivering vaginally was .54 and for those delivered surgically .50. The mean number of prenatal risks for the same two subgroups were .36 and .62, respectively. The reasons cited for surgical intervention were, in order of frequency, dystocia and cephalopelvic disproportion (31 percent), repeat c-section (22 percent), fetal distress (15 percent), breech presentation (11 percent), labor not progressing (9 percent), medical conditions contraindicating vaginal delivery (diabetes, herpes, toxemia) (5 percent), hemorrhagic conditions (abruptio placentae, placenta previa) (4 percent), premature and/or

TABLE 3. Number of Mothers Reporting Health-Related Problems during Pregnancy

Problem	Hospital Mothers ($N = 402$)	Center Mothers ($N = 100$)	Home Mothers ($N = 100$)
Aches or pains	279 (69%)	62	66
Asthma or allergy	32 (8)	23	10
Cardiovascular problems	79 (20)	14	5
Cold or cough	261 (65)	58	56
Constipation	135 (34)	32	27
Diarrhea	40 (10)	19	16
Edema	206 (51)	55	41
Eyes or ears	33 (8)	4	13
Fever	56 (14)	15	10
Gastrointestinal problems	216 (54)	62	60
Infection, systemic	73 (18)	17	12
Infection, vaginal	121 (30)	34	23
Nausea or vomiting	229 (57)	61	59
Nervousness, anxiety	60 (15)	7	7
Sleep	168 (42)	42	37

TABLE 4. Percentage of Prenatal Risks Occurring in More than 1 Percent of Each Group, as Reported by Health Personnel

Hospital Mothers (N = 402)		Center Mothers (N = 100)		Home Mothers (N = 100)	
Risk	Occurrence	Risk	Occurrence	Risk	Occurrence
Preeclampsia	44%	Vaginal spotting	5%	Post term	4%
Chronic hypertension	20	Uterine-cervical abnormality	3	Vaginal spotting	3
Diabetes	17	Post term	2	Previous premature birth	2
Abnormal fetal position	11			Viral infection	2
Endometritis	7				
Multiple pregnancy	7				
Post term	7				
Vaginal spotting	7				
Intrauterine growth retardation	6				
Viral infection	5				

TABLE 5. Percentage of Intrapartal Risks Occurring in More
than 1 Percent of Each Group, as Reported by Health Personnel

Hospital Mothers ($N = 402$)		Center Mothers ($N = 100$)		Home Mothers ($N = 100$)	
Risk	Occurrence	Risk	Occurrence	Risk	Occurrence
Electronic fetal monitor[a]	19%	none		none	
Heavy meconium	13				
Premature rupture of membranes	3				
Shoulder dystocia	2				

[a]Category includes bradycardia (16 percent), tachycardia, decreased baseline variability, late decelerations, variable decelerations, and fetal distress.

prolonged rupture of membranes (3 percent), and prolapsed umbilical cord (less than 1 percent).

The mean number of health-related problems reported by Hospital, Center, and Home Mothers, respectively, were 5.25 (SD = 1.78), 4.84 (SD = 2.23), and 5.43 (SD = 2.50). These means are not significantly different [$F(2,588) = 2.29$]. Table 3 shows a breakdown of health-related problems in terms of the number of mothers who reported experiencing each of the fifteen during their pregnancies. There is little apparent difference in the relative frequencies: regardless of group, mothers were most apt to experience aches and pains, gastrointestinal upsets, and nausea or vomiting in connection with their pregnancies as well as at least one cold or coughing spell during the nine-month period. The only real difference among groups was in terms of the number of mothers reporting bouts of asthma or allergy [$X^2(2) = 18.81$, $p < .0001$] and cardiovascular problems [$X^2(2) = 12.88$, $p < .002$].

The picture of similarities gives way to one of differences when one looks at the strategies these women used in coping

with their health-related problems. The mean probability that
mothers would choose to treat their problems through some
form of drug therapy was .38 (SD = .25), .38 (SD = .26),
and .23 (SD = .26) for Hospital, Center, and Home
Mothers, respectively. The difference among these means is
highly significant: $F(2,591) = 14.72$, $p < .0001$. Looking at
the number of mothers who chose to treat their symptoms
with drugs (table 6) reveals that Hospital and Center Mothers
were very similar in the frequency and pattern of resort to
drug therapy. It also indicates that Home Mothers were consistently less inclined than Hospital and Center Mothers to
use drug therapy. In their interviews, Home Mothers repeatedly mentioned doing nothing or using nondrug alternatives
as a first step in their therapeutic strategies, e.g., elevating
their feet for edema; munching dry soda crackers for morning
sickness.

TABLE 6.   Number of Mothers Resorting to Drug Therapy

Problem	Hospital Mothers	Center Mothers	Home Mothers
Aches or pains	126 (45%)	34 (55%)	20 (30%)
Asthma or allergy	20 (63)	9 (39)	3 (30)
Cardiovascular problems	15 (19)	0 (0)	0 (0)
Cold or cough	144 (55)	38 (66)	19 (34)
Constipation	51 (38)	8 (25)	5 (18)
Diarrhea	15 (38)	4 (21)	2 (12)
Edema	5 (2)	2 (4)	0 (0)
Eyes or ears	9 (27)	0 (0)	2 (15)
Fever	29 (52)	10 (67)	0 (0)
Gastrointestinal problems	118 (55)	33 (53)	14 (23)
Infection, systemic	63 (86)	14 (82)	10 (83)
Infection, vaginal	101 (84)	29 (85)	12 (52)
Nausea or vomiting	60 (26)	15 (25)	8 (14)
Nervousness, anxiety	9 (15)	2 (24)	1 (14)
Sleep	8 (5)	0 (0)	1 (3)

Note: Percentages based on figures in table 3.

Drug-Taking Patterns during Pregnancy

Table 7 shows the number of mothers who consumed differing numbers of drugs. The distributions for Hospital Mothers and Center Mothers are strikingly similar, whereas both are dissimilar to the pattern of drug consumption for Home Mothers, 42 percent of whom took no drugs at all. This divergence is statistically significant: $X^2(12) = 58.64$, $p < .0001$. On the average, Hospital Mothers consumed 2.34 (SD = 1.98) drugs, Center Mothers consumed 2.47 (SD = 2.17) drugs, and Home Mothers consumed 1.12 (SD = 1.31) prenatal drugs.

Combining all groups, 602 mothers consumed a total of 122 different drug products which contained 154 different ingredients. A breakdown by groups shows that the total number of different drug products (and ingredients) consumed by Hospital Mothers was 100 (129); by Center Mothers, 56 (81); and by Home Mothers, 37 (69). Prescription products accounted for 34 percent of the drugs consumed by Hospital Mothers, 38 percent of the drugs consumed by Center Mothers, and 30 percent of those consumed by Home Mothers.

The most frequently consumed drug products are shown in table 8. Most heavily represented are analgesics (aspirin and Tylenol, the single most popular drug with all groups); antacids (Rolaids, Maalox, Alka Seltzer, Mylanta, Tums, Digel);

TABLE 7. Number of Mothers Consuming Drugs during Pregnancy

Number of Drugs	Hospital Mothers ($N = 402$)	Center Mothers ($N = 100$)	Home Mothers ($N = 100$)
None	56 (14%)	18	42
1 or more	346 (86)	82	58
2 or more	240 (60)	59	29
3 or more	152 (38)	42	14
4 or more	84 (21)	25	5
5 or more	57 (14)	15	3
6 or more	29 (7)	13	1

TABLE 8. The Ten Most Frequently Consumed Prenatal Drugs

Hospital Mothers		Center Mothers		Home Mothers	
Drug	% Consuming	Drug	% Consuming	Drug	% Consuming
Tylenol	36.32	Tylenol	48.00	Tylenol	17.00
Rolaids	9.70	Maalox	16.00	Tums	7.00
ampicillin	8.40	Mylanta	14.00	aspirin	6.00
Bendectin	8.21	Sudafed	13.00	Bendectin	4.00
aspirin	7.71	Bendectin	12.00	Monistat	4.00
Sudafed	6.97	ampicillin	11.00	Rolaids	3.00
Maalox	6.72	Monistat	10.00	Afrin	2.00
Robitussin	5.47	aspirin	7.00	Digel	2.00
Summer's Eve	4.98	Mycostatin	7.00	ampicillin	2.00
Massengill douche	4.78	Robitussin	6.00	Robitussin	2.00

Note: These tabulations required information about the specific drug product consumed. Vitamins were not included because a pilot study revealed that women, on the whole, regarded vitamins as a class rather than as a group of individual drug products. Ingredients for the drug products listed in this table can be found in table 14.

cough/cold remedies (Sudafed, Robitussin, Afrin); and antiinfectives (ampicillin, Monistat, Mycostatin). Vitamins were not counted as drugs in this tally. Most of the most popular drugs are nonprescription products. The outstanding exception is Bendectin, a prescription product used for its antiemetic properties. Bendectin was among five most consumed drugs for all groups. (In 1983, the manufacturer of Bendectin announced that it was being withdrawn from the market in response to the growing number of product liability suits brought against it.)

Correlational analyses were performed to examine the relationships between number of drugs consumed and other variables of interest. The procedure used here and elsewhere was justified on the basis of the normality of residuals from the regression model. These analyses showed a strong association between prenatal drug consumption and number of health-related complaints within each of the three groups: Hospital Mothers ($r = .62, p < .0001$), Center Mothers ($r = .50, p < .0001$), and Home Mothers ($r = .43, p < .0001$). Considering Hospital Mothers only, higher prenatal drug consumption was associated with increasing age ($r = .21, p < .0001$), amount of information about teratogenic drugs in general ($r = .32, p < .01$), and exposure to sources of information about drugs ($r = .15, p < .003$).

Table 9 shows the numbers and percentages of mothers in each group who consumed differing numbers of products containing caffeine, alcohol, tobacco, or marijuana. Hospital Mothers lead in reported consumption of caffeinated products and cigarettes but not in consumption of alcoholic beverages and marijuana, where Center Mothers report higher intakes. Home Mothers are consistently restrained in their use of all products.

Patterns of Drug Administration during Childbirth

Table 10 shows the number of mothers who received drugs during childbirth. Medication-free delivery occurred in 97 per-

TABLE 9. Number of Mothers Consuming Druglike Products (caffeine, alcohol, cigarettes, and marijuana) during Pregnancy

Product	1. Hospital Mothers	2. Center Mothers	3. Home Mothers	X^2 1 vs 2 vs 3 (df = 2)	2 vs 3 (df = 1)
Coffee (cups/day)				20.40***	7.85**
0	239 (59.4%)	68	85		
1 or more	163 (40.6)	32	15		
Tea (cups/day)				39.99***	NS
0	174 (43.3)	67	74		
1–2	142 (35.3)	23	19		
3 or more	86 (21.4)	10	7		
Soft drinks/day				65.43***	NS
0	193 (48.0)	83	83		
1 or more	209 (52.0)	17	17		
Beers/week				10.48**	NS
0	366 (91.0)	80	91		
1 or more	36 (9.0)	20	9		
Wine (glasses/week)				45.24***	6.66*
0	384 (95.5)	74	89		
1 or more	18 (4.5)	26	11		
Mixed (drinks/week)				NS	NS
0	380 (94.5)	98	100		
1 or more	22 (5.5)	2	0		
Cigarettes/day				25.83***	NS
0	272 (67.7)	83	91		
1 or more	130 (32.3)	17	9		
Marijuana/week				24.29***	NS
0	384 (95.5)	81	91		
1 or more	18 (4.5)	19	9		

*$p \leq .01$ **$p \leq .005$ ***$p \leq .0001$

TABLE 10. Number of Mothers to Whom Drugs Were Administered during Labor and Delivery

Number of Drugs	Hospital Mothers (N = 402)	Center Mothers (N = 100)	Home Mothers (N = 100)
0	6 (1.5%)	72	97
1 or more	396 (98.5)	28	3
2 or more	374 (93.0)	12	2
3 or more	333 (82.8)	4	0

cent of home deliveries, 72 percent of center deliveries, but less than 2 percent of hospital deliveries. None of the Home Mothers received more than two drugs intrapartally, whereas 9 percent of the Hospital Mothers received at least two. The diversity in these patterns of obstetric drug consumption was highly significant $[X^2(2) = 430.36, p < .0001]$ in comparing medication-free to medicated deliveries.

The average number of drugs administered was 4.97 (SD = 2.60) for Hospital Mothers, .47 (SD = .90) for Center Mothers, and .05 (SD = .30) for Home Mothers. The overall difference among means is significant: $F(2,582) = 298.84$, $p < .0001$. Duncan follow-up tests showed that Center and Home Mothers did not differ significantly in obstetric drug administration. Hospital Mothers, however, were administered significantly more obstetric drugs than both out-of-hospital groups.

For all groups combined, the total number of different drug products administered was fifty-eight, which represented sixty-two different drug ingredients. All fifty-eight were administered to Hospital Mothers. Center Mothers received seven different products, and Home Mothers, three.

The drugs most frequently administered during labor and delivery are shown in tables 11 and 12. Whereas the most frequently consumed prenatal drugs are largely over-the-counter products, the drugs most frequently administered during labor and delivery are largely prescription products. Functionally, most are administered as analgesics or anesthetics.

Correlational analyses showed that for Hospital Mothers there were significant associations between low intrapartal drug intake and high obstetric drug information ($r = -.13$, $p < .009$), fewer prenatal and obstetric risks ($r = .22$, $p < .0001$), and more childbirth experiences ($r = -.14$, $p < .007$). For Center Mothers as well, the association between low intrapartal drug exposure and previous childbirth experiences was significant ($r = -.34$, $p < .001$).

TABLE 11. Number of Mothers Exposed to Drugs Most Frequently Administered during Labor and Delivery

Hospital Mothers (N = 402)			Center Mothers (N = 100)			Home Mothers (N = 100)		
dextrose 5%/.2% sodium chloride	326	81.1%	hydroxyzine hydrochloride	17	17%	oxytocin	2	2%
oxytocin	158	39.3	meperidine hydrochloride	15	15	magnesium sulfate	1	1
nitrous oxide	130	32.3	promethazine hydrochloride	6	6	meperidine hydrochloride	1	1
succinylcholine chloride	124	30.8	dextrose 5%/.2% sodium chloride	1	1			
promethazine hydrochloride	118	29.4	naloxone hydrochloride	1	1			
tubocurarine chloride	115	28.6	oxytocin	1	1			
meperidine hydrochloride	113	28.1						
Maalox aluminum hydroxide magnesium hydroxide	101	25.1						
sodium thiopental	90	22.4						
lidocaine hydrochloride	86	21.4						

Note: Drugs are listed by generic name. For brand name equivalents, see App. B.

TABLE 12. Functional Grouping of Drugs Most Frequently
Administered during Labor and Delivery

Drug	Number of Mothers Receiving
Premedication Agents	
Uterine stimulants	161
oxytocin (Pitocin)	
Products ancillary to administration of other drugs	327
and intervention procedures	
dextrose 5%/.2% sodium chloride	
Narcotic analgesics	128
meperidine hydrochloride (Demerol)	
Narcotic antagonists	1
naloxone hydrochloride (Narcan)	
Tranquilizers	141
hydroxyzine hydrochloride (Vistaril)	
promethazine hydrochloride (Phenergan)	
Antacids	101
aluminum hydroxide, magnesium hydroxide (Maalox)	
Anesthetics and Related Agents	
Neuromuscular blocking agents	239
tubocurarine chloride (curare)	
succinylcholine chloride (Anectine)	
Local anesthetics	86
lidocaine hydrochloride (Xylocaine)	
Inhalant anesthetics	130
nitrous oxide	
Intravenous anesthetics	90
sodium thiopental (Pentothal)	

Rx for Mothers Equals Risk for Babies?

One of the main concerns of this study was safety for the fetus
of the drugs consumed by their mothers. Drug "safety" is
traditionally indexed as absence of empirically demonstrable
adverse fetal effects following prenatal, perinatal, or neonatal
exposure to the drug. Although the exposure may come about
through direct administration, it is generally indirect, through
administration to the pregnant or nursing mother. The term
adverse fetal effects is defined as evidence of toxicity, structural
teratogenicity, or behavioral teratogenicity.

Proof that a drug is safe for human consumption before it can be marketed for human consumption was required for the first time in 1938, when Congress passed the Federal Food, Drug, and Cosmetic Act. In this act, Congress charged the Food and Drug Administration (FDA) with responsibility for approving each new prescription drug as safe before allowing the manufacturer to distribute it for clinical use.[9] Any such approval by the FDA is not an across-the-board one, however. Approval is restricted to those specific purposes which the manufacturer named in its new drug application and for which the manufacturer supplied the FDA with data documenting the prescription drug's safety. Once approval has been obtained and the drug has entered the domain of clinical use, medical personnel may begin to use it for purposes other than those originally approved. When an approved drug is used for such a nonapproved purpose, it is technically held to be an "experimental drug" once again (U.S. Food and Drug Administration 1972).

The question naturally arises, how safe for their offspring were the drugs consumed by the mothers in this study? Four different approaches were used in attempting to answer this question. First, we asked how many of the prescription products consumed by our 602 respondents had actually been approved by the FDA as safe for use during pregnancy or labor and delivery. To do this, we examined the descriptive statements on the printed inserts included in the packaging of the drugs. Package insert statements are written by the drug manufacturer and edited by the FDA. For most drugs, these

---

9. In 1962, Congress amended the Food, Drug, and Cosmetic Act to require that drugs be proven effective as well as safe. However, our concern is with potential adverse effects on the fetus, and thus is limited to safety. Drug effectiveness is a logical impossibility for the fetus since it is but an incidental recipient of the drug consumed by its mother for her health-related problems.

Two things should be noted about the empirical data involved in the FDA's assessment of safety. First, they are gathered by the manufacturer of the experimental drug, not by the FDA or by an independent agency. Second, they are never made available to public scrutiny even after the drug has been approved and distributed for clinical use.

statements are available not just as printed pieces of paper in the package itself but are also published in the annually issued *Physicians Desk Reference* (commonly referred to as "PDR"). In some cases, the package insert was unclear or uninformative with respect to safe use during pregnancy and childbirth. For these cases, we requested clarification or information directly from the FDA.

The results of this review of the FDA approval are shown in table 13. As that table reveals, among all the drugs actually administered during labor and delivery, 47 (89 percent) have apparently never been approved by FDA as safe for use for that purpose. The number of drugs (six) actually approved by the FDA was about the same as the number of drugs (five) not approved but used anyway.

Among the drugs most frequently administered during labor and delivery (see table 11), only one (meperidine) has been approved by the FDA for use during labor and delivery. The breakdown by group is as follows. Of the ten drugs most frequently used in hospital delivery, nine were prescription drugs: one (meperidine) has been approved by the FDA for use in labor and delivery; two (succinylcholine and lidocaine) are unclear with respect to approval status; and six have apparently not been approved. Of the six drugs most frequently used in delivery at the birth center, one (meperidine) has been approved by the FDA as safe for use in labor and delivery, and five have not. Of the three drugs most frequently used in home delivery, one (meperidine) has been approved by the FDA as safe for use during labor and delivery, and two have not.

Our second approach in attempting to assess the extent to which the drugs consumed by the mothers in this study were safe for their unborn babies was to determine, for each drug, whether empirical studies on adverse fetal effects have actually been carried out and published in the scientific research literature. To this end, we carried out a nonevaluative literature review for each of the ingredients contained in all drug prod-

TABLE 13.   Safety of Drugs Used during Labor and Delivery

	Status of FDA Approval for Safe Use			
Prescription Drug	Approved	Not Approved	Unclear	No Information
alphaprodine hydrochloride	+			
aminophylline				+
ampicillin				+
atropine sulfate				+
bupivacaine hydrochloride	+			
butorphanol tartrate	+			
chloroprocaine hydrochloride			+	
clindamycin hydrochloride				+
codeine sulfate				+
cortisone acetate				+
cyclobenzaprine				+
dexamethasone				+
dextrose 5%/.2% sodium chloride				+
diazepam		+		
digoxin				+
dimenhydrinate				+
diphenhydramine hydrochloride				+
ephedrine				+
epinephrine				+
erythromycin				+
fentanyl		+		
furosemide				+
gentamicin				+
halothane				+
heparin sodium				+
hydralazine hydrochloride				+
hydroxyzine hydrochloride				+
isoxsuprine hydrochloride				+
ketamine		+		
lidocaine hydrochloride			+	
magnesium sulfate				+
meperidine hydrochloride	+			
metaproterenol sulfate				+
methoxyflurane	+			
methylprednisolone				+
methylprednisolone sodium succinate				+
morphine sulfate			+	
naloxone				+
nitrous oxide				+
oxytocin				+
pancuronium bromide	+			

TABLE 13—*Continued*

Prescription Drug	Status of FDA Approval for Safe Use			
	Approved	Not Approved	Unclear	No Information
penicillin				+
pentobarbital		+		
phenobarbital				+
potassium chloride				+
prochlorperazine				+
promethazine hydrochloride				+
propranolol				+
ritodrine hydrochloride				+
sodium thiopental				+
succinylcholine chloride			+	
tretracaine hydrochloride		+		
tubocurarine chloride				+

Note: Drugs are listed by generic name. For brand name equivalents, see App. B.

ucts represented in this study. (Some drug products contain more than one ingredient.) The complete results of this review are in tables 14 and 15. The literature search made use of Medline computerized data base for the years 1976–83 as well as four comprehensive reviews of the literature to locate studies published before 1976.

We included in the review all studies in which the design allowed for tests of statistical significance and also allowed evaluation of the contribution of single agents to adverse effects. In other words, we did not include studies in which the effects of two or more agents were inextricably confounded, e.g., a study not allowing separation of the effects of butorphanol and meperidine was not included.

The 602 women in our sample reported consuming 122 different drug products with 154 different ingredients during pregnancy. We found no published reports of safety or lack of it for 71 percent of these drug ingredients.

A total of fifty-eight different drug products with sixty-two different ingredients was administered intrapartally to the 602

TABLE 14. Documented Adverse Effects of Drug Products Consumed Prenatally

Drug Product[a] (P = Prescription)	Studies of Ingredients Documenting Adverse Effects[b]	Studies of Ingredients Finding No Adverse Effects[b]	Ingredients for Which No Published Studies Were Found
Aci-Jel Therapeutic Vaginal Jelly (P)			acetic acid oxyquinoline sulfate ricinoleic acid boric acid glycerin
Actifed (P)	pseudoephedrine hydrochloride (237)	pseudoephedrine hyrochloride (115)	triprolidine hydrochloride
Afrin			oxymetazoline hydrochloride sorbitol glycine sodium hydroxide sodium bicarbonate citric acid
Alka-Seltzer	aspirin (22, 26, 33, 49, 52, 66, 68, 80, 87, 131, 132, 139, 141, 157, 160, 163, 173, 180, 181, 183, 192, 208, 221, 236, 253, 256, 262, 268, 284, 290)	aspirin (33, 141, 239, 264)	
Alka-Seltzer Plus	aspirin (supra)	aspirin (supra)	chlorpheniramine phenylpropanolamine bitartrate
Allerphen (P) aminophylline (P) ampicillin (P)	aminophylline (34) ampicillin (38, 209)		chlorpheniramine maleate
Anacin	aspirin (supra) caffeine (2, 20, 24, 53, 69, 97, 152, 207, 213, 229)	aspirin (supra) caffeine (33, 158, 283)	

Anbesol			phenol benzocaine glycerin
aspirin	iodine (11)		
Asthma Nefrin	aspirin (supra) epinephrine hydrochloride (27, 29, 36, 45, 63, 79, 106, 115, 125, 126, 134, 142, 162, 168, 187)	aspirin (supra)	chlorobutanol
AVC Cream (P)	sulfanilamide (110)	sulfanilamide (211)	allantoin aminocrine hydrochloride
Azogantrisin (P)	sulfisoxazole (211)		
BC Powder	aspirin (supra) salicylamide (128) caffeine (supra)	aspirin (supra) caffeine (supra)	potassium chloride
Benadryl (P)	diphenhydramine hydrochloride (15, 42, 123, 178)	diphenhydramine hydrochloride (93, 116)	
Bendectin (P)	Bendectin (252, 285)	doxylamine succinate (102)	pyridoxine hydrochloride
Betadine	povidone-iodine (241)		

Note: As a result of government reviews of OTC products, formulations of some drugs are changing. This table reflects as accurately as possible the formulation at the time the study was performed. Alcohol as an ingredient was not included since exposure was to a minute quantity used as a vehicle for other ingredients.

[a]All drugs were administered orally, intravenously, intramuscularly, or subcutaneously except those administered topically, indicated as (T).

[b]See App. C for numbered references to studies cited.

TABLE 14—*Continued*

Drug Product[a] (P = Prescription)	Studies of Ingredients Documenting Adverse Effects[b]	Studies of Ingredients Finding No Adverse Effects[b]	Ingredients for Which No Published Studies Were Found
Bicozene Cream			benzocaine resorcin
Black Draught			senna anise clove peppermint cinnamon magnesium carbonate aluminum glycinate
Bufferin	aspirin (supra)		phenol
Chloraseptic Throat Spray			sodium phenolate
Chlor-Trimeton Choledyl (P) Chooz	ephedrine sulfate (237)	ephedrine sulfate (115)	chlorpheniramine maleate oxtriphylline magnesium trisilicate calcium carbonate
Clomid (P)	clomiphene citrate (9, 28, 77, 94, 117, 156, 193)	clomiphene citrate (124, 289)	
Colace			dioctyl sodium sulfosuccinate
Comtrex	acetaminophen (236)	acetaminophen (290)	dextromethorphan hydrobromide chlorpheniramine maleate phenylpropanolamine hydrochloride

Product		
Contac	chlorpheniramine maleate phenylpropanolamine hydrochloride	
Coricidin-D	aspirin (supra)	chlorpheniramine maleate phenylpropanolamine hydrochloride
Correctol		dioctyl sodium sulfosuccinate yellow phenolpthalein
CoTylenol	phenylephrine hydrochloride (38, 138) acetaminophen (supra)	chlorpheniramine maleate
Creomulsion		acetaminophen (supra)
		creosote ipecac white pine menthol cascara wild cherry beechwood
Darvocet (P)	acetaminophen (supra) propoxyphene napsylate (37, 81)	acetaminophen (supra) propoxyphene napsylate (127)
Darvon (P)	propoxyphene hydrochloride (supra)	propoxyphene hydrochloride (supra)
Datril	acetaminophen (supra)	acetaminophen (supra)
Demerol (P)	meperidine hydrochloride (118, 226, 245, 258, 270, 273)	meperidine hydrochloride (233)

TABLE 14—*Continued*

Drug Product[a] (P = Prescription)	Studies of Ingredients Documenting Adverse Effects[b]	Studies of Ingredients Finding No Adverse Effects[b]	Ingredients for Which No Published Studies Were Found
Desitin			zinc oxide talc petrolatum lanolin cod liver oil
Dicarbosil			calcium carbonate peppermint oil
Di-Gel			aluminum hydroxide magnesium oxide simethicone
Dramamine	dimenhydrinate (30)		
Dristan	phenylephrine hydrochloride (supra) aspirin (supra) caffeine (supra)	aspirin (supra) caffeine (supra)	magnesium carbonate aluminum hydroxide phenidamine tartrate
Excedrin	aspirin (supra) salicylamide (supra) caffeine (supra) acetaminophen (supra)	aspirin (supra) caffeine (supra) acetaminophen (supra)	
Excedrin PM	pyrilamine maleate (198) acetaminophen (supra)	pyrilamine maleate (14) acetaminophen (supra)	
Ex-Lax			yellow phenolpthalein

Product	Ingredients
FDS (T)	isopropanol myristate mineral oil lanolin yellow phenolphthalein methylene chloride (218, 251, 267)
Feen-A-Mint	
Flagyl (P)	metronidazole (39, 65)
Fleet Enema	sodium biphosphate sodium phosphate
Fletcher's Castoria	senna
Flexeril (P)	cyclobenzaprine
Gantrisin (P)	sulfisoxazole (supra)
Garamycin (P)	gentamicin
Gaviscon	magnesium trisilicate sodium bicarbonate alginic acid aluminum hydroxide
Gelusil	aluminum hydroxide magnesium hydroxide simethicone
Haley's M-O	magnesium hydroxide mineral oil
Halls Mentholyptus Cough Drops	menthol eucalyptus oil
heparin sodium (P)	heparin sodium
Hiprex (P)	methenamine hippurate
Inderal (P)	propranolol hydrochloride (1, 3, 18, 222, 224, 232) propranolol hydrochloride (85)

TABLE 14—Continued

Drug Product[a] (P = Prescription)	Studies of Ingredients Documenting Adverse Effects[b]	Studies of Ingredients Finding No Adverse Effects[b]	Ingredients for Which No Published Studies Were Found
insulin	insulin (8, 82, 91, 111, 129, 148, 150, 154, 205)	insulin (6, 44, 199, 201)	
Kaopectate			kaolin pectin
Keflex (P)			cephalexin
Librium (P)	chlordiazepoxide hydrochloride (280, 286)		
Lomotil (P)	atropine sulfate (212)	atropine sulfate (99)	diphenoxylate
Maalox			aluminum hydroxide magnesium hydroxide
Massengill Disposable Douche			cetylpyridinium chloride lactic acid octoxynol
magnesium sulfate	magnesium sulfate (54, 279)		
Metamucil			psyllium mucilloid
Metaprel (P)			metaproterenol sulfate
Milk of Magnesia			magnesium hydroxide peppermint oil
Monistat (P)			miconazole
Mycolog (P)	triamcinalone acetonide (175, 206, 228, 235, 260, 272)		nystatin neomycin sulfate gramicidin
Mycostatin (P)			nystatin

Mylanta	magnesium hydroxide aluminum hydroxide simethicone
Neo-Synephrine	phenylephrine hydrochloride (supra)	benzalkonium chloride
Norforms Novacain (P) Novahistine		methylbenzethonium chloride procaine hydrochloride chlorpheniramine maleate phenylpropanolamine hydro- chloride
Nyquil	acetaminophen (supra) ephedrine sulfate (supra)	acetaminophen (supra) doxylamine succinate (supra) ephedrine sulfate (supra)

Parapectolin	paregoric (15, 46, 72, 78, 84,
	  86, 88, 98, 105, 144, 145,
	  188)
		pectin
		kaolin

penicillin (P) Pepto-Bismol Percogesic Peri-Colace	penicillin (15, 92) bismuth subsalicylate (112) acetaminophen (supra)	penicillin (120, 161) bismuth subsalicylate (202) acetaminophen (supra) calcium carbonate phenyltoloxamine citrate casanthranol dioctyl sodium sulfosuccinate

Phenergan (P)	promethazine hydrochloride
	  (96, 180)
		promethazine hydrochloride
		  (93)

Phenergan Expectorant with
  Codeine (P)
	promethazine hydrochloride
	  (supra)
	codeine phosphate (15, 72)
		promethazine hydrochloride
		  (supra)
		potassium guaicolsulfonate
		citric acid
		sodium citrate

phenobarbital (P)	phenobarbital (58, 61, 64, 119, 122, 130, 160, 190, 250)	

TABLE 14—*Continued*

Drug Product[a] (P = Prescription)	Studies of Ingredients Documenting Adverse Effects[b]	Studies of Ingredients Finding No Adverse Effects[b]	Ingredients for Which No Published Studies Were Found
Phiso-Derm (T)			entsufon sodium petrolatum lanolin cholesterols
prednisone (P)	prednisone (95, 215, 289)		
Preparation H (T)			shark liver oil live yeast extract phenylmercuric nitrate
Primatene Mist	epinephrine hydrochloride (supra)		
Pristeen (T)			cetearyl octonate isopropanol myristate
Privine Nose Drops			naphazoline hydrochloride benzalkonium chloride
progesterone (P)	progesterone (13, 249)	progesterone (32, 133, 197, 214, 242, 259, 266)	
Riopan			magaldrate
Robitussin			guaifenesin
Robitussin DM			dextromethorphan hydrobromide guaifenesin

Product			
Rolaids			dihydroxyaluminum sodium carbonate
secobarbital (P)			
Sine-Off	secobarbital (17, 21) aspirin (supra)	aspirin (supra)	chlorpheniramine maleate, phenylpropanolamine hydrochloride
Sinutab	acetaminophen (supra)	acetaminophen (supra)	phenylpropanolamine hydrochloride, phenyltoloxamine citrate
Sudafed	pseudoephedrine hydrochloride (supra)	pseudoephedrine hydrochloride (supra)	
Sultrin Cream (P)	sulfathiazole (203)		sulfacetamide, sulfabenzamide, sodium citrate, citric acid, zinc sulfate, allantoin
Summer's Eve			
Tegrin (T)			coal tar extract
Theo Dur (P)	theophylline (76, 97)		
Triaminic Syrup	pyrilamine maleate (supra)	pyrilamine maleate (supra)	phenylpropanolamine hydrochloride, pheniramine maleate, calcium carbonate, peppermint oil
Tums			
Tylenol	acetaminophen (supra)	acetaminophen (supra)	

TABLE 14—*Continued*

Drug Product[a] (P = Prescription)	Studies of Ingredients Documenting Adverse Effects[b]	Studies of Ingredients Finding No Adverse Effects[b]	Ingredients for Which No Published Studies Were Found
Tylenol #3 (with codeine) (P)	codeine phosphate (supra) acetaminophen (supra)	acetaminophen (supra)	
Vagisil			benzocaine resorcin allantoin aminocrine hydrochloride
Vagitrol (P)	sulfanilamide (supra)	sulfanilamide (supra)	
Valium (P)	diazepam (113, 147, 155, 165, 171, 174, 182, 248, 280)	diazepam (35, 149, 248, 280)	
Vasocon-A (P)			naphazoline hydrochloride antazoline phosphate phenylmercuric acetate sodium chloride sodium carbonate boric acid
Vasodilan (P) Va-Tro-Nol	isoxsuprine hydrochloride (83) methyl salicylate (4, 40, 57, 100, 230) ephedrine sulfate (supra)	ephedrine sulfate (supra)	menthol eucalyptol camphor
Velosef (P)			cephradine

Product		
Vicks Formula 44	doxylamine succinate (supra)	dextromethorphan hydrobromide
		sodium citrate
Vicks Vapo Rub (T)		camphor
		menthol
		turpentine spirits
		eucalyptus oil
		cedar leaf oil
		myristica oil
		thymol
Visine (T)		tetrahydrozaline
Vistaril (P)	hydroxyzine hydrochloride (121, 172)	

TABLE 15. Documented Adverse Effects of Drug Products Administered Intrapartally

Drug Product[a] (P = Prescription)	Studies of Ingredients Documenting Adverse Effects[b]	Studies of Ingredients Finding No Adverse Effects[b]	Ingredients for Which No Published Studies Were Found
Alupent (P)			metaproterenol sulfate
aminophylline (P)	aminophylline (34)		
ampicillin (P)	ampicillin (38, 209)		
Anectine (P)			succinylcholine chloride
Apresoline (P)			hydralazine hydrochloride
atropine sulfate (P)	atropine sulfate (212)	atropine sulfate (99)	
Benadryl (P)	diphenhydramine hydrochloride (15, 42, 123, 178)	diphenhydramine hydrochloride (93, 116)	
Cleocin (P)		clindamycin hydrochloride (196)	
codeine sulfate (P)	codeine sulfate (15, 72)		
Colace			dioctyl sodium sulfosuccinate
Compazine (P)	prochlorperazine (37, 195)	prochlorperazine (194)	
cortisone acetate (P)	cortisone acetate (10, 12, 31, 41, 48, 55, 60, 70, 89, 90, 137, 151, 189, 215)	cortisone acetate (228)	
curare (P)	tubocurarine hydrochloride (23, 67, 71)		
Decadron (P)	dexamethasone (281, 282, 288)	dexamethasone (28)	
Demerol (P)	meperidine hydrochloride (118, 226, 245, 258, 270, 273)	meperidine hydrochloride (233)	

dextrose 5% in 0.2% sodium chloride solution (P)			
digoxin (P)	dextrose (254, 258)		digoxin
Dramamine		dimenhydrinate (30)	
ephedrine sulfate (P)	ephedrine sulfate (237)	ephedrine sulfate (115)	
epinephrine (P)	epinephrine (27, 29, 36, 45, 63, 79, 106, 115, 125, 126, 134, 142, 162, 168, 187)		
erythromycin (P)	erythromycin (47)		cyclobenzaprine
Flexeril (P)			gentamicin
Garamycin (P)			
halothane (P)	halothane (19, 50, 59, 74, 101, 135, 140, 159, 167, 185, 244, 257)	halothane (269)	
heparin sodium (P)			heparin sodium
Inderal (P)	propranolol hydrochloride (1, 3, 18, 222, 232)	propranolol hydrochloride (85)	
insulin	insulin (8, 82, 91, 111, 129, 148, 150, 154, 205)	insulin (6, 44, 199, 201)	
ketamine hydrochloride (P)			ketamine hydrochloride
Lasix (P)			furosemide
lidocaine hydrochloride (P)	lidocaine hydrochloride (107, 108, 143, 210, 217, 225)		

Note: As a result of government review of OTC products, formulations of some drugs are changing. This table reflects as accurately as possible the formulation at the time the study was performed. Alcohol as an ingredient was not included since exposure was to a minute quantity used as a vehicle for other ingredients.

[a] All drugs were administered orally, intravenously, intramuscularly, subcutaneously, or by inhalation.

[b] See App. C for numbered references to studies mentioned.

TABLE 15—*Continued*

Drug Product[a] (P = Prescription)	Studies of Ingredients Documenting Adverse Effects[b]	Studies of Ingredients Finding No Adverse Effects[b]	Ingredients for Which No Published Studies Were Found
Maalox			aluminum hydroxide magnesium hydroxide
magnesium sulfate (P)	magnesium sulfate (54, 279)		
Marcaine (P)	bupivacaine hydrochloride (191)	bupivacaine hydrochloride (62, 184, 204)	
Medrol (P)	methylprednisolone (same as cortisone acetate supra)		
Milk of Magnesia			magnesium oxide peppermint oil
morphine sulfate (P)	morphine sulfate (46, 78, 84, 86, 88, 98, 105, 144, 145, 188)		
Narcan (P)			naloxone hydrochloride
Nembutal (P)	pentobarbital (61, 104, 153, 186, 200)		
Nesacaine (P)		chloroprocaine hydrochloride (204)	
Nisentil (P)	alphaprodine hydrochloride (276)		
nitrous oxide (P)	nitrous oxide (5, 7, 16, 56, 114, 146, 169, 170, 220, 234, 271)	nitrous oxide (291)	
oxytocin (P)	oxytocin (51, 75, 103, 176, 191, 216, 223, 238, 240, 255, 261)	oxytocin (164, 166, 179, 227, 231, 247, 267, 277)	

Pavulon (P)		pancuronium bromide
penicillin (P)	penicillin (15, 92)	penicillin (120, 161)
Penthrane (P)	methoxyflurane (25, 219)	methoxyflurane (43)
Pentothal (P)	sodium thiopental (73, 109)	sodium thiopental (136)
Phenergan (P)	promethazine hydrochloride (96, 180)	promethazine hydrochloride (93)
phenobarbital (P)	phenobarbital (58, 61, 64, 119, 122, 130, 160, 190, 250)	
potassium chloride (P)		potassium chloride
ritodrine hydrochloride (P)		ritodrine hydrochloride (274, 275)
Solu-Medrol (P)	methylprednisolone sodium succinate (see cortisone acetate supra)	
Stadol (P)		butorphanol tartrate
Sublimaze (P)		fentanyl
tetracaine hydrochloride (P)		tetracaine hydrochloride
Tylenol	acetaminophen (236)	acetaminophen (290)
Valium (P)	diazepam (113, 147, 155, 165, 171, 174, 182, 248)	diazepam (35, 149)
Vasodilan (P)	isoxsuprine hydrochloride (83, 243)	
Vistaril (P)	hydroxyzine hydrochloride (121, 172)	

women in our sample. We found no published reports regarding safety for 33 percent of these drug ingredients.

None of the ten ingredients contained in five of the ten drugs most frequently consumed by Hospital Mothers during pregnancy (see table 8) has been studied regarding adverse effects on the fetus. These drugs and their unstudied ingredients are Rolaids (dihydroxyaluminum sodium carbonate), Maalox (aluminum hydroxide and magnesium hydroxide), Robitussin (guaifenesin), Summer's Eve (sodium citrate, citric acid, and zinc sulfate), and Massengill douche (cetylpyridinium chloride, lactic acid, and octoxynol). There were also five drugs in which none of the ingredients has been studied in the list of the ten drugs consumed most frequently by Center Mothers during pregnancy (see table 8). These include Maalox (aluminum hydroxide and magnesium hydroxide), Mylanta (magnesium hydroxide, aluminum hydroxide, and simethicone), Monistat (miconazole), Mycostatin (nystatin), and Robitussin (guaifenesin). Of the ten most frequently consumed prenatal drugs by Home Mothers (see table 8), six consist entirely of ingredients that have not been studied. These include Tums (calcium carbonate and peppermint oil), Monistat (miconazole), Rolaids (dihydroxyaluminum sodium carbonate), Afrin (oxymetazoline hydrochloride, sorbitol, glycine, sodium hydroxide), Digel (aluminum hydroxide, magnesium oxide, simethicone), and Robitussin (guaifenesin).

Two of the ten products most frequently administered intrapartally to Hospital Mothers (see table 11) consist entirely of ingredients that have never been studied. These drug products and their ingredients are Anectine (succinylcholine chloride), and Maalox (aluminum hydroxide and magnesium hydroxide). Center Mothers were administered six different drugs during labor and delivery (see table 11). Of these six, only one drug product, Narcan (naloxone hydrochloride) has not been studied. Home Mothers were administered three different drugs during labor and delivery. These three drugs have been studied.

Our third approach to the question of safe drug use in

pregnancy, labor, and delivery was to review and summarize
those studies that have actually been carried out and published in the scientific literature. The resulting summaries are
shown in table 16 (for prenatal exposure) and table 17 (for
perinatal exposure).

Of the one hundred drug products which Hospital Mothers
reported consuming during their pregnancies, fifty-two contain
one or more ingredients which are implicated in adverse effects. Of the 402 Hospital Mothers in this study, 64 percent
consumed at least one drug so implicated; 29 percent, two or
more; 11 percent, three or more; 4 percent, four or more.
Center Mothers reported consuming fifty-six different drug
products prenatally, twenty-eight of which contain at least one
ingredient which is implicated in adverse effects. At least one
drug so implicated was consumed by 68 percent of the 100
Center Mothers in our sample; two or more by 35 percent,
three or more by 14 percent, and four or more by 2 percent.
Sixteen of the thirty-seven drug products that Home Mothers
reported consuming during their pregnancies contain one or
more ingredients implicated in adverse effects. Of these 100
women, 38 percent consumed at least one drug so implicated;
6 percent, two or more; and 2 percent, three. (None of the
Home Mothers took more than three implicated drugs.)

Of the fifty-eight different drugs administered to Hospital
Mothers during labor and delivery, thirty-six have been implicated as having adverse effects. Of the 402 mothers who de-

TABLE 16. Number of Mothers Prenatally Consuming Drugs
with Research-Documented Teratogenic or Toxic Effects

Number of Drugs	Hospital Mothers ($N = 402$)	Center Mothers ($N = 100$)	Home Mothers ($N = 100$)
none	145 (36%)	32	62
1 or more	257 (64)	68	38
2 or more	118 (29)	35	6
3 or more	44 (11)	14	2
4 or more	16 (4)	2	0

TABLE 17. Number of Mothers Intrapartally Consuming Drugs
with Research-Documented Teratogenic or Toxic Effects

Number of Drugs	Hospital Mothers (N = 402)	Center Mothers (N = 100)	Home Mothers (N = 100)
none	12 (3.0%)	72	97
1 or more	390 (97.0)	28	3
2 or more	346 (86.1)	13	2
3 or more	267 (66.4)	3	0

livered in-hospital, 97 percent received at least one of these
drugs; 86 percent at least two; and 66 percent at least three.
Center Mothers received a total of six different obstetric drugs,
five of which have been implicated as having adverse effects. Of
the 100 Center Mothers in our study, 28 percent received at
least one of these drugs; 13 percent at least two; and 3 percent
at least three. Home Mothers received three different obstetric
drugs. All three drugs have been implicated as having adverse
effects. Of these 100 women, 3 percent received at least one of
these drugs and 2 percent received two. (None of the women in
this group took more than two of these drugs.)

Tables 13–17 relate the literature on adverse effects of
mothers' actual drug consumption. For prenatal drug use,
there is a highly significant difference between groups in terms
of the number of mothers who consumed no drug implicated
by the research literature as teratogenic or toxic and those who
consumed one or more such drugs: $X^2(2)$ = 25.46, p < .0001.
For intrapartal drug use, the between-group differences are
even more striking: $X^2(2)$ = 436.91, p < .0001.

The fourth method used in assessing drug safety was directed exclusively toward nonprescription or over-the-counter
(OTC) products, which constituted the bulk of prenatally consumed drugs. As with prescription drugs, the FDA bears responsibility for clearing nonprescription products on the
grounds of safety before they are released for marketing.
However, whereas prescription products need only be safe for
particular, specified uses, OTC products must be found safe
for general use and safe for use in doses larger than those

recommended. OTC product labels must also indicate precautions or limits to their safe application. In the late 1970s, the state of California and consumer groups throughout the country began to express their concern about these labels, in particular about their failure to include cautionary statements to potential consumers who are pregnant or nursing. In the fall of 1982, after several hearings on the matter, the FDA proposed amending the general provisions for all systemically absorbed OTC drugs to require that their package labels contain the following warning: "As with any drug, if you are pregnant or nursing a baby, seek professional advice before using this product." The regulation became effective December 3, 1982, although drug manufacturers were permitted to defer labeling changes for a year thereafter.

How many of the systemically absorbed products consumed by mothers in this study included cautionary statements on their labels? The present authors investigated this by examining labeled information on the exterior packaging of these products, all of which were available at local pharmacies. This "research" was carried out in the spring of 1983, five months after the FDA had begun requiring (but also deferring) labeling changes and six months after the state of California had begun requiring labeling changes (a move that caused many manufacturers to change labels destined for all interstate shipments). We found that while twenty products contained cautionary statements directed to pregnant or nursing women, over 2.5 times as many (fifty-two) contained no word of warning at all. The authors updated this "research" in January, 1984, and found that only forty-one of the same products contained cautionary statements to pregnant or nursing women. The remaining thirty-one products contained no such warning and were, therefore, in violation of the FDA regulation over a year after it had become effective. Almost none of the products in the antacid, laxative, and antidiarrheal categories conformed with the labeling regulation; almost all the products in the analgesic and cold and cough preparations categories did conform with the labeling regulation.

Mothers' Information about Drugs

A major focus of concern in this investigation was the knowledge that mothers had about the drugs they consumed during pregnancy, labor, and delivery. Mothers were questioned about each of these drugs in terms of the nine points of information recommended for consumers by the American Society of Hospital Pharmacists and the U.S. Pharmacopoeia (table 18). Their responses were scored positively for correct information and negatively for misinformation. Hence, scores ranged from a possible +9 through −9. Mean prenatal drug information scores were obtained by averaging across all drugs reportedly consumed during pregnancy, and mean intrapartal drug information scores by averaging across all drugs administered during labor and delivery. Vitamins were included in analyzing the informational variables.

Information about Drugs Consumed Prenatally

Table 18 shows the number of mothers who had information about the drugs they consumed during their pregnancies. As these data indicate, most mothers knew the names of the drugs they took and the actions they expected them to have. Most Center and Home Mothers also knew the dosage and administration schedules. Beyond that, information dropped sharply. Less than 10 percent of any group was aware of the potential for adverse effects.

Table 18 also shows that Home Mothers were better informed on every point than either of the other two groups. Similarly, Center Mothers were better informed than Hospital Mothers, with the exception of one point (self-monitoring techniques). These differences are reflected in the mean prenatal drug information scores for the three groups: 1.58 (SD = .66) for Hospital Mothers, 2.66 (SD = .88) for Center Mothers, and 3.22 (SD = 1.41) for Home Mothers. The overall differences are highly significant: $F(2,567) = 164.36, p < .0001$. The mean

TABLE 18.   Mothers' Information about Drugs Consumed during
Pregnancy

| Items of Consumer Information | Number of Informed Mothers[b] | | |
	Hospital (N = 386)	Center (N = 98)	Home (N = 96)
1. Name of drug	245 (63.5%)	88 (89.8%)	92 (95.8%)
2. Drug's intended use, expected action	215 (55.7)	74 (75.5)	82 (85.4)
3. Administration: route, dose, schedule	138 (35.8)	66 (67.3)	76 (79.2)
4. Special directions for preparation, administration	10 (2.6)	8 (8.2)	29 (30.2)
5. Precautions	2 (0.5)	4 (4.1)	10 (10.4)
6. Adverse effects of drug	5 (1.3)	5 (5.1)	8 (8.3)
7. Self-monitoring techniques	1 (0.2)	0	8 (8.3)
8. Contraindications, including drug/drug and drug/food interactions	4 (1.0)	4 (4.1)	10 (10.4)
9. Misc., including missed dose, prescription refill information, etc.	3 (0.8)	3 (5.1)	16 (16.7)

[a]From the American Society of Hospital Pharmacists
[b]All Ns based on number of women consuming one or more prenatal products, including vitamins.

information score for prescription drugs was 3.29 (SD = .76) and that for nonprescription drugs, 2.69 (SD = .85).

Correlational analyses showed, as the strongest relationships, that Hospital Mothers who were more informed about prenatal drugs were also more informed about the intrapartal drugs they received ($r = .33$, $p < .0001$), were more often in contact with sources of information about drugs ($r = .20$, $p < .0001$), engaged in more health-promoting behaviors ($r = .29$, $p < .0001$), and perceived themselves as being in control of their environments, i.e., internally oriented locus of control ($r = -.34$, $p < .0001$). In addition, Hospital Mothers who were more informed about prenatal drugs were older ($r = .17$, $p < .0009$), better educated ($r = .29$, $p < .0001$), and more apt to be white than nonwhite ($r = .21$, $p < .0001$).

Within the Center and Home groups, more prenatal drug

information was associated with more information about teratogenic drugs in general (Center: $r = .26$, $p < .01$; Home:
$r = .36$, $p < .0006$) and with greater participation in health-
promoting behaviors (Center: $r = .23$, $p < .03$; Home: $r = .32$, $p < .002$). Those Center Mothers who had relatively more
prenatal risk factors also tended to have more prenatal drug
information ($r = .28$, $p < .009$).

Information about Intrapartal Drugs

The mean intrapartal drug information score was .29 (SD =
.45) for Hospital Mothers and 2.42 (SD = 1.00) for Center
Mothers. (A mean for Home Mothers was not calculated because the Ns involved were too small: three Home Mothers
consumed four drugs.) The difference between these two
means was highly significant: $t(418) = 10.82$, $p < .0001$. There
was also a significant difference between prenatal and intra-
partal drug information scores for Hospital Mothers [$t(378) = 37.91$, $p < .0001$], but not for Center Mothers [$t(24) = 2.36$, $p < .01$], indicating that Hospital Mothers knew even less about
their obstetric medications than they did about their prenatal
medications. In fact, most Hospital Mothers had no information about the drugs administered to them during labor and
delivery. For example, 98 percent could not name the drugs
they had received, and 96 percent were not aware they received one or more drugs administered to them.
    Correlational analyses showed that, for Hospital Mothers,
information about intrapartal drugs was significantly related to
information about drugs consumed prenatally. It was also related to several other variables. Hospital Mothers who were
more informed about drugs administered intrapartally consumed fewer such drugs ($r = -.13$, $p < .009$). They were also
more informed about teratogenic drugs in general ($r = .38$, $p < .002$), as were Center Mothers ($r = .58$, $p < .003$), were
more often in contact with sources of information ($r = .15$, $p < .003$), and engaged in more health-promoting behaviors (r

= .16, p < .002). Additionally, Hospital Mothers who were relatively more informed about intrapartally administered drugs were more likely to be white (r = .22, p < .0001) and were better educated (r = .22, p < .0001).

Information about Drugs in General

Incorporated into the interview was a twelve-item test designed to assess the amount of information mothers had about teratogenic drugs in general, irrespective of any differences in their medical conditions that may have required medication. The items consisted of twelve drugs documented in the research literature as teratogens: six drugs commonly administered during labor and delivery and six more frequently administered for other conditions. Responses were scored by using a relevant subset (four points of information) of the nine points of information recommended for consumers by the American Society of Hospital Pharmacists (1976).

Table 19 contains the basic data on mothers' information about drugs in general. The overall between-group difference in information was highly significant [$F(2,251)$ = 42.89, p < .0001], although this significance is attributable to the difference between Hospital Mothers and the other two groups, whose information scores were essentially the same.

As noted previously, Center and Home Mothers who were better informed about teratogenic drugs in general also knew more about the drugs they had consumed prenatally. Those Hospital and Center Mothers having relatively more information about the intrapartal drugs they received were also more knowledgeable about teratogenic drugs in general. Hospital Mothers who knew more about teratogenic drugs in general were older (r = .35, p < .004), better educated (r = .48, p < .0001), and white (r = .38, p < .0003). More information about teratogenic drugs within the Home group was associated with higher education (r = .38, p < .0001) and greater participation in health-promoting behaviors (r = .36, p < .0005).

TABLE 19. Results of Test on Information about Drugs Documented in Research Literature as Teratogens

Test Items	Mean Information Score[b]		
	Hospital Mothers (N = 65)	Center Mothers (N = 96)	Home Mothers (N = 92)
Drugs Commonly Used in Obstetrics[a]			
alphaprodine hydrochloride (Nisentil)	−0.02	0.48	0.42
hydroxyzine hydrochloride (Vistaril)	0.06	0.54	0.44
lidocaine hydrochloride	0.02	0	0
meperidine hydrochloride (Demerol)	0.12	1.00	0.84
nitrous oxide	0.02	0.23	0.12
promethazine hydrochloride (Phenergan)	0.05	0.43	0.20
Overall Mean	0.12	0.65	0.62
Drugs Commonly Used outside Obstetrics[a]			
amphetamine	1.03	3.44	3.39
aspirin	1.83	3.31	3.93
caffeine	1.09	3.05	3.14
diethylstilbestrol (DES)	0.68	1.78	2.33
phenytoin sodium (Dilantin)	0.46	1.72	2.24
propoxyphene hydrochloride (Darvon)	0.40	1.25	1.07
Overall Mean	0.79	2.22	2.36

[a]Drug Information Service, University of Florida
[b]Possible scores range from −4 (completely incorrect information) to +4 (completely correct information)

Finally, mothers were asked whether they would like more information about drugs should they again become pregnant. An affirmative response to this question was given by 72 percent of Hospital Mothers, 41 percent of Center Mothers, and 45 percent of Home Mothers. Chi-square analysis showed that these proportions are significantly different: $X^2(2) = 53.66$, $p < .0001$.

Sources of Information

Whenever a respondent reported having taken a drug (or refrained from having taken one), and had indicated how much information she had about that drug, she was also asked where she had gotten information about that drug. Specifically, she was asked whether any of the following had served as sources of information: acquaintance, friend, or relative; magazine or newspaper; package label; pharmacist; physician; television; other source.

Table 20 presents data on sources of information about specific drugs. These data show the relative frequency with which mothers mentioned these sources of information. Thus, for example, Hospital Mothers cited an acquaintance, friend, or relative as having provided information about a specific drug on ninety-three occasions. As the data indicate, physician and clinic nurses ("other") were, for Hospital Mothers, the most frequently cited sources of information about specific drugs. For Center and Home Mothers, the most frequently cited sources of information were midwives and printed reference material ("other").

Later in the interview, each mother was asked to rank the same sources of information in the order that she relied on them for information about medications in general, assigning a "1" to the source she relied upon most, a "2" to the next most relied upon source, etc. These data are shown in table 21, in which the entries indicate the percentage distribution of rankings by each group for each source of information about drugs

TABLE 20.   Sources of Information about Specific Drugs by
Number of Times Cited

Source	Hospital Mothers	Center Mothers	Home Mothers
Acquaintance, friend, or relative	93 (7.1%)	35 (9.0%)	61 (15.7%)
Magazine or newspaper	8 (0.6)	7 (1.8)	28 (7.2)
Package label	108 (8.3)	15 (3.9)	41 (10.6)
Pharmacist	9 (0.7)	1 (0.2)	1 (0.2)
Physician	490 (37.6)	32 (8.3)	50 (12.9)
Television	17 (1.3)	6 (1.6)	4 (1.0)
Other[a]	577 (44.3)	291 (75.2)	203 (52.3)
Total citations	1,302	387	388

Note: Entries are number of times each source was cited as having provided information about a specific drug.

[a]For Hospital Mothers, "other" most often referred to clinic nurse. For Center and
Home Mothers, "other" most often referred to midwives and next most often referred to
written materials such as books and articles.

in general. For instance, 9.9 percent of Hospital Mothers relied most on an acquaintance, friend, or relative for drug information, while 13.7 percent of Home Mothers cited this
source as the one most frequently used.

Table 22 compares sources of information about specific
drugs which mothers actually consumed (or refrained from
consuming) (see table 20) with sources of information about
medications in general (see table 21). The two rankings agree
rather closely. In only one case (Center Mothers/Pharmacist)
is there a discrepancy of as much as three ranks.

Also relevant to an understanding of where and how
mothers obtain their information about drugs were individual
interview questions asking about exposure to information:
whether mother had read any books on childbirth; whether
such books contained information about drugs; whether she
had attended childbirth education classes; whether the curricu-
lum had included drugs as a topic; and whether, during her
pregnancy, she had discussed the question of drugs with a

TABLE 21. Sources of Information about Drugs in General

Source	Rank (1 = source most relied on)						
	1	2	3	4	5	6	7
Acquaintance, friend, or relative							
Hospital mothers	9.9%	16.9%	22.9%	20.1%	14.8%	14.1%	1.3%
Center mothers	9.9	15.7	22.4	19.3	15.3	15.4	2.0
Home mothers	13.7	14.7	17.9	17.9	16.8	16.8	2.2
Magazine or newspaper							
Hospital mothers	3.0	4.8	12.6	26.1	35.5	17.2	0.8
Center mothers	3.2	5.4	10.8	26.1	35.1	17.6	1.8
Home mothers	5.4	11.8	12.9	26.9	22.6	15.1	5.3
Package label							
Hospital mothers	5.1	9.8	32.4	26.9	14.1	11.2	0.5
Center mothers	5.1	10.5	33.2	28.2	13.1	9.2	0.7
Home mothers	8.5	21.3	26.6	19.2	14.9	9.5	0
Pharmacist							
Hospital mothers	7.4	51.4	18.9	9.4	7.6	3.9	1.4
Center mothers	8.0	48.4	21.8	9.7	7.2	3.5	1.4
Home mothers	6.5	23.9	23.9	18.5	16.3	7.6	3.3

Note: Entries indicate the percentage distribution of rankings for each source. Example: 9.9 percent of hospital subjects who ranked the source acquaintance, friend, or relative assigned it a rank of 1. Each row sums to 100 percent.

TABLE 21—*Continued*

| Source | \multicolumn{7}{c}{Rank (1 = source most relied on)} | | | | | | |
	1	2	3	4	5	6	7
Physician							
Hospital mothers	72.7%	13.4%	7.8%	2.5%	3.0%	0.6%	0%
Center mothers	62.0	17.5	9.0	4.0	4.2	1.9	1.4
Home mothers	28.1	20.8	16.7	11.5	11.5	7.3	4.1
Television							
Hospital mothers	2.7	3.8	3.8	12.4	23.5	48.6	5.2
Center mothers	2.3	2.8	3.6	9.9	21.7	46.7	13.0
Home mothers	2.2	1.1	1.1	5.6	15.7	41.7	32.6
Other							
Hospital mothers	17.5	19.3	14.0	7.0	7.0	8.8	26.4
Center mothers	44.0	13.8	7.3	4.1	4.6	3.7	22.5
Home mothers	59.7	16.1	3.2	1.6	1.6	0	17.8

TABLE 22. Rank Ordered Comparison Showing Frequency of Citation of Drug Information Sources

	Hospital Mothers		Center Mothers		Home Mothers	
	Specific (N = 402)	General (N = 395)	Specific (N = 100)	General (N = 98)	Specific (N = 100)	General (N = 96)
Acquaintance, friend, or relative	4	3	2	3	2	3
Magazine or newspaper	7	6	5	6	5	6
Package label	3	5	4	5	4	4
Pharmacist	6	4	7	4	7	5
Physician	2	1	3	1	3	2
Television	5	7	6	7	6	7
Other	1	2	1	2	1	1

Source: Based on data from tables 20 and 21.

TABLE 23. Other Sources of Information about Drugs

Interview Question	Hospital Mothers (N = 402)	Center Mothers (N = 100)	Home Mothers (N = 100)
Read books, articles on pregnancy and delivery?	72.9%	96.0%	98.0%
Contain information on medications?	58.8	80.2	88.4
Attend childbirth education classes?	31.2	96.0	80.5
Include information on medications?	64.8	74.0	78.6
Did your doctor discuss medications with you?	45.5	36.0	24.7

physician. Table 23 summarizes mothers' responses to these questions.

As the data in table 23 indicate, almost all Center and Home Mothers availed themselves of written material about childbirth, whereas less than three-fourths of the Hospital Mothers did so. Intergroup differences were even larger when the content of the reading material addressed itself to drugs. Similarly, almost all Center Mothers attended childbirth education classes, whereas less than one-third of Hospital Mothers and only 80 percent of Home Mothers did so. These differences are in large part attributable to the fact that attendance was required for Center Mothers and that most of the Center Mothers were primiparous whereas most of the Hospital and Home Mothers were multiparous. Although relatively few of the Center and Home Mothers used the services of a physician, all Hospital Mothers did so. Nevertheless, less than half of the Hospital Mothers reported that their doctors had provided them with information about drugs.

Individual Difference Variables

Each Mother completed the Rotter Locus of Control Scale (Rotter 1966) for the purpose of assessing the extent to which she perceived herself as being in control of her environment as opposed to being controlled by that environment. Mean scores for Hospital Mothers ($N = 181$), Center Mothers ($N = 95$), and Home Mothers ($N = 88$) were 11.49 (SD = 4.11), 9.28 (SD = 3.93), and 7.86 (SD = 4.25), respectively. Analysis of variance revealed a highly significant between-group difference: $F(2,351) = 23.95$, $p < .0001$.

As previously noted, locus of control was significantly associated in Hospital Mothers with information about drugs consumed during pregnancy. Locus of control was also related to other variables. Hospital Mothers who perceived themselves as being in control also exposed themselves to more sources of information ($r = -.22$, $p < .003$) and engaged in more health-promoting behaviors ($r = -.28$, $p < .0001$). They also tended to be older ($r = -.27$, $p < .002$) and better educated ($r = -.24$, $p < .002$).

The twenty-five-item Health-Promoting Behavior Scale, incorporated into the interview, measured the extent to which mothers actually did exercise control over factors known to promote health and prevent disease, e.g., use of seat belts, avoidance of smoking, maintenance of proper weight for height, etc. Mean scores for Hospital, Center, and Home Mothers were 85.87 (SD = 8.72), 95.05 (SD = 8.31), and 95.76 (SD = 6.86), respectively. These means are significantly different: $F(2,598) = 86.38$, $p < .0001$.

As mentioned above, engagement in health-promoting behaviors was related to more information about drugs consumed prenatally, more information about intrapartal drugs, more information about teratogenic drugs in general, and an internal locus of control within the various groups as described previously. Within the Hospital and Home groups, participation in more health-promoting behaviors was associated with exposure to more sources of information (Hospital: $r = .31$, $p < .0001$; Home: $r = .34$, $p < .0007$). Home Mothers who engaged in more health-promoting behaviors experienced fewer health-related complaints prenatally ($r = -.26$, $p < .01$). Older women within the Hospital and Center groups engaged in more health-promoting behaviors (Hospital: $r = .14$, $p < .005$; Center: $r = .26$, $p < .008$) and for all three groups, greater participation in health-promoting behaviors characterized better-educated women (Hospital: $r = .45$, $p < .0001$; Center: $r = .32$, $p < .002$; Home: $r = .38$, $p < .0001$).

CHAPTER 5

A Closer Look at the Findings

This study investigated maternal drug consumption and infant drug exposure during pregnancy and childbirth, the status of those drugs with respect to adverse fetal effects, and the amount of information mothers have about the drugs they have consumed.

Subjects were 602 mothers who delivered clinically normal babies. Of the total, 402 had chosen to deliver in-hospital ("Hospital Mothers"); 100, at a freestanding birth center ("Center Mothers"); and 100, at home ("Home Mothers").

Data on drug consumption and drug information were obtained by interview and from medical records. Drug information was scored according to consumer information standards recommended by the American Society of Hospital Pharmacists.

The three groups of mothers did not differ in the number of health-related problems they reported experiencing during their pregnancies. However, Hospital Mothers significantly exceeded Center and Home Mothers in resorting to drugs as the therapy of choice in coping with those problems. During pregnancy, Hospital and Center Mothers consumed significantly more prescription drugs, nonprescription drugs, and druglike products than did Home Mothers. During childbirth, significantly more drugs were administered to Hospital Mothers than to Center or Home Mothers.

Four approaches were used in assessing drug safety, defined as the absence of empirically demonstrated adverse fetal effects. First, inquiries revealed that most of the drugs actually

administered during labor and delivery had never been approved for that purpose by the FDA. Second, a literature
search revealed no published reports of safety (or lack of it)
for two-thirds of the prenatally consumed drug ingredients and
one-third of the intrapartally administered drug ingredients.
Third, for those drugs for which there are published reports,
more than half of the drugs consumed or administered contain
one or more ingredients implicated by empirical study as having adverse effects on the fetus. Fourth, a check of pharmacy
shelves revealed over two-thirds of nonprescription products
consumed carried no labeled cautionary warning directed to
pregnant women.

    Finally, the data indicated that, in general, mothers know
very little about the drugs they consume during pregnancy and
even less about the drugs administered to them during childbirth. Home Mothers were significantly better informed than
Center Mothers who, in turn, were significantly better informed than Hospital Mothers.

    These findings will now be discussed in greater detail.

Participant Profiles

Table 2 (see chap. 4) contains basic demographic information
on the three groups of mothers. The profile for each group is
distinctive. Most Hospital Mothers were multiparas. Their
average age was 22.7 years. For the nation as a whole, between the years 1975 and 1979, the average age of mothers at
time of birth of their first child was 22.3 years (U.S. Bureau of
the Census 1982). Hospital Mothers had completed 11.3 years
of education, 1 year less than the 1981 average for the United
States (Bureau of the Census 1982), 3+ years less than Center
Mothers, and 2+ years less than Home Mothers. Hospital
Mothers were also less advantaged than Center Mothers and
Home Mothers in terms of need for financial aid and minority
representation. They were traditional in religious affiliation
but not in family structure: in more than 40 percent of cases,

Hospital Mothers would return with their babies to fatherless homes.

By way of contrast, the typical Center Mother in this study was primiparous and had postponed motherhood longer than usual for females in the United States. These socioeconomically advantaged women, for the most part, were college-educated, employed outside the home, and white. Their babies would become members of nuclear families traditional in every respect except religious affiliation.

The demographic characteristics of Center Mothers in this study were similar to those of other American women currently choosing to deliver at freestanding birth centers. Reports indicate that most such mothers are married, well educated, gainfully employed, upper middle class, white, and twenty-five years or older when they first become mothers.[10]

The profiles for Hospital and Center Mothers were not only different from each other but each was distinct from that characterizing Home Mothers. Most Home Mothers were multiparous. Of the seventy-one multiparas, sixty had also had their previous child out-of-hospital. As a group, they were more socioeconomically heterogeneous than their Hospital or Center counterparts. They were strongly traditional in family structure and strongly nontraditional in religious ties. The profile of Home Mothers in this study is similar to that for home birth mothers throughout the United States, according to NAPSAC statistics[11] and according to the findings of Herman, Miller-Klein, and Ventre (1979).

According to the latter sources, most home birth couples are white, married, and middle-class. They have some college education; they are gainfully employed in white collar, profes-

10. Diony Young, personal communication, January, 1984. See also R. L. Cohen, A comparative study of women choosing two different childbirth alternatives, *Birth* 9 (1982): 13–23.

11. Dr. David Stewart, personal communication, January, 1984. NAPSAC stands for InterNational Association of Parents and Professionals for Safe Alternatives in Childbirth.

sional, or technical capacities; their combined income is greater than the national average; they own their home and at least one car. Home birth mothers are in their early twenties when their first child is born and in their late twenties when their second child is born.

The main purpose of the study did not include an assessment of mothers' reasons for choosing one birthplace over another. Nevertheless, we did attempt to estimate this for a subsample of twenty-four Center Mothers and twenty-four Home Mothers whom we reinterviewed briefly by telephone to ask why they had chosen to birth out-of-hospital and what they saw as the relative risks involved in in-hospital birth as opposed to out-of-hospital birth. The great majority (75 percent) of these respondents were of the opinion that in-hospital birth was as risky or riskier than out-of-hospital birth, citing, as documentation for their beliefs, the high probability of infection; enforced mother-child separation; and "being pressured into accepting excessive interventions," especially drugs, induced and augmented labor, and surgical delivery (Brackbill, Rice, and Young 1984). Nevertheless, Center Mothers most frequently cited safety as a principal reason for choosing center over home as a place of birth, whereas Home Mothers frequently cited cost as a major reason in choosing home over center. Home Mothers also frequently cited the psychological advantages of home as a place of birth, noting that birth at home is a warm, natural, family-oriented, controllable experience.

Health Problems and Risks

Although these groups were very different in demographics, they were indistinguishable in terms of self-reported, health-related complaints occurring during pregnancy (table 3, chap. 4). Some of these problems were frequent concomitants of pregnancy, e.g., edema; others simply happened to occur during pregnancy, e.g., colds; all have in common that they were relatively mild in symptomatology and short-lived in nature.

In sharp contrast to the between-group similarities in health-related complaints are the large between-group differences in prenatal and intrapartal risks reported by health personnel (tables 4 and 5, chap. 4). The most notable difference among the prenatal risks was the diagnosis of "pre-eclampsia," noted in 44 percent of the medical records of Hospital Mothers. At the University of Florida's Shands Hospital, this diagnosis is based on the simultaneous occurrence of edema, high blood pressure, and protein in the urine. In conjunction with this point, it should be pointed out that Shands is a referral hospital so that risks are truly overrepresented among its obstetrical patients. On the other hand, each of the three components of the diagnosis depends, to some degree, on subjective judgment.

The most striking between-group difference in risk occurred as the result of using electronic fetal monitoring, which, according to the consistent findings of previously published research, leads to greater numbers of "high risk" determinations and hence to greater numbers of surgical deliveries. (For reviews of electronic fetal monitoring and its attendant problems, see Banta and Thacker 1979; Brackbill, Rice, and Young 1984; International Childbirth Education Association 1981). Surgical delivery was indeed the outcome for 37 percent of Shands's obstetrical patients during the period of data collection. (Mothers delivered surgically were overrepresented in this study because they remained in the hospital longer than mothers delivering normally and were therefore more apt to be available as interviewees.)

Drug Remedies

For all groups combined, mothers consumed an average of 2.16 drugs during their pregnancies. This figure is lower than those reported by other investigators. For example, in an earlier study of mothers delivering at Shands Hospital, Doering and Stewart (1978) reported an average prenatal drug consumption of 11.0. It is unlikely that the lower figure reported here represents a decreasing trend in drug consumption during pregnancy (Brackbill 1979, 89). Rather, it is most probably attributable to methodological differences in data collection. In the Doering and Stewart study, as well as others focusing exclusively on drug consumption, mothers have been asked to keep daily diary accounts of drug intake or have been interviewed repeatedly during their pregnancies. In the present study, investigators interviewed mothers only once, in an interview that covered the entire nine-month period of pregnancy.

A lower figure for prenatal drug intake probably also reflects the fact that most of the products consumed prenatally in this study were over-the-counter (OTC) products, and OTC products are often not thought of as "drugs" or "medications" (see Woodward et al. 1982, 169). The same belief has been targeted for comment in other studies (e.g., Hill 1973), although the extent to which it abounds is not known. The misapprehension that nonprescription drugs are not real drugs is addressed below in regard to drug safety.

Considering the three groups separately, it was noted earlier that there were highly significant differences among groups in prenatal drug consumption, Home Mothers consuming, on the average, less than half the number of drugs consumed by Hospital Mothers and Center Mothers (who used equal numbers of drug products). It was also noted that although there were no differences among groups in number of health-related complaints, there were highly significant associations between prenatal drug consumption and number of health-related complaints for all groups. The association was strongest ($r = .62$) for Hospital Mothers and least strong ($r = .43$) for Home Mothers, who often reported trying a nondrug remedy as first therapeutic choice.

In the consumption of druglike products (caffeine, alcohol, tobacco, and marijuana), Home Mothers were again relatively more abstemious. Center Mothers, who were similar to Hospital Mothers in the consumption of "real" drugs, were more similar to Home Mothers in the consumption of druglike products, with the result that the biggest differences in the latter category were between Hospital Mothers and the other two groups. Although there was no source of external validation for consumption of druglike products, there was also no reason to suspect that one group would be more prone than another to favor social acceptability over candor in their responses.

Turning to obstetric drugs, we found striking differences among groups in the administration of intrapartal medication: an average of 4.97 drugs for Hospital Mothers, 0.47 for Center Mothers, and 0.05 for Home Mothers. The percentage of medication-free deliveries among Hospital Mothers was less than the percentage of medicated deliveries among Home Mothers (table 10, chap. 4). Hospital Mothers received fifty-eight different drug products; Center Mothers, seven; and Home Mothers, three. Anesthetic agents, which figured prominently in hospital deliveries, were entirely absent in center and home deliveries. For Hospital Mothers, obstetrical drug administration was modestly though significantly related to prenatal risk factors ($r = .23$, $p < .0001$), as determined by health personnel.

Drug Safety

A major purpose of this study was to investigate the safety to infants of the drugs to which they were incidentally exposed prenatally and perinatally. "Safety" was defined as the absence of adverse fetal effects or, more concretely, as empirical evidence failing to find toxicity, structural teratogenicity, or behavioral teratogenicity. Results indicated the following.

- Of the 154 different ingredients consumed during pregnancy, a search of the literature revealed no studies relating to safety in 71 percent of cases.

- Of the ten drugs most frequently used by Hospital Mothers during their pregnancies (table 8, chap. 4), a literature search indicates that five consist of ingredients whose safety has apparently never been evaluated, and that three of the remaining five show evidence of adverse fetal effects more often than evidence of safety.

- At least one drug with documented adverse effects was consumed prenatally by 64 percent of Hospital Mothers, by 68 percent of Center Mothers, and by 38 percent of Home Mothers. Since 71 percent of the drug ingredients mothers consumed during pregnancy have apparently never been studied, our results must underestimate the actual extent of teratogenic exposure.

- Of the nonprescription products consumed by mothers in this study, 72 percent had apparently been marketed without labeled warning directed toward the pregnant or nursing consumer. Results of an update, conducted more than a year after an FDA regulation requiring such labeling became effective, revealed that 43 percent of these products still contained no labeled warning and were, therefore, in violation of that regulation. Antacid, laxative, and antidiarrheal products violated this regulation most frequently while analgesics and cough and cold preparations violated this regulation least frequently.

- Of the fifty-three prescription drugs administered during labor and delivery only six, or 11 percent, have actually been approved by the FDA as safe for use for that purpose (table 13, chap. 4). The remaining 89 percent have apparently either never been considered by the FDA or never been cleared by that agency as nonproductive of adverse fetal effects.

- Of the six drugs approved by the FDA as safe for use during childbirth, a review of the literature shows more evidence of adverse fetal effects than evidence of safety in the case of three drugs (alphaprodine or Nisentil; meperidine or Demerol; methoxyflurane or Penthrane) and no evidence at all regarding safety in the case of two other drugs (butorphanol or Stadol and pancuronium bromide or Pavulon).[12]

- Among the ten drugs most frequently administered in hospital obstetrics (table 11, chap. 4) only one (meperidine) has been approved by the FDA as safe for use for that purpose. Nevertheless, there are in the scientific literature more studies showing adverse fetal effects of meperidine than there are studies showing no adverse fetal effects.

- Among the remaining nine drugs most frequently administered in hospital obstetrics, two (succinylcholine and Maalox) consist entirely of ingredients whose safety for the fetus has apparently never been evaluated, while the other seven are linked in the scientific literature to adverse fetal effects more often than to safety.

- At least one drug with documented adverse fetal effects was administered intrapartally to 97 percent of Hospital Mothers. At least two such drugs were administered to 86 percent of Hospital Mothers, and at least three to 66 percent of Hospital Mothers.

Animal Research: An Important Contribution

Having summarized the evidence relating to safety or lack of it, some comments are now in order on the nature of that evidence. One important aspect to consider regarding studies of drug teratogenicity, as summarized in tables 14 and 15 (chap. 4), is that most of the studies have been carried out on animals. This is because it is extremely difficult, if not impossible, to establish that an agent is teratogenic solely through

---

12. Recall that the data on the basis of which FDA determines safety are not those carried out in independent laboratories and published subject to peer review, in the mainstream of the scientific literature. They are (1) provided by the drug manufacturer and (2) never made available for inspection by persons outside the employ of the FDA or drug manufacturer.

observational or epidemiological studies of human beings. Experimental, animal studies are essential. Nevertheless, one may still ask whether it is valid to generalize from animal research to the human situation.

Both as scientists and laypersons, we tend to judge the admissibility of animal research by shifting standards. On the one hand, we agree with the FDA requirement that every experimental drug be tested on animals prior to its being tested on humans and that it be discarded if it produces teratogenic changes in those test animals. On the other hand, we sometimes find ourselves in situations where we are less accepting of animal research. For example, large numbers of habitual consumers of soft drinks sweetened with saccharin protested attempts to generalize from rats to human beings with regard to carcinogenicity potential.

Yet, if animal research isn't generalizable, why do scientists bother doing it? And why does society condone, promote, or even insist on animal research? Ethics provide one reason. For at least fifteen centuries, since the time of Galen, mankind has held that it is not morally admissible to conduct risky experimentation on human beings in the absence of animal data allowing estimation of that risk. So strongly held is this ethical principle that its violation predictably elicits public outrage and retaliation. For example, under the Nazi regime, German physicians' extensive human biomedical experimentation (Mitscherlich and Mielke 1949) led to their being tried as war criminals as well as to formulation of the first ethical code specifying ground rules for experimentation on human subjects (Permissible medical experiments, n.d.; see also Ivy 1948). Of this code's ten guidelines, the third states categorically that human experimentation must be based on the results of animal experimentation indicating a high probability that "the anticipated results will justify the performance of the experiment" (*Trials of War Criminals* 1949, 181–82). In other words, the Nuremberg Code is unequivocal in its position that we not only can generalize from animals to humans but must do so.

A second reason why science acknowledges the applicability to humans of animal data stems from the logical consideration that mammals share many fundamental biological similarities, including basic aspects of reproductive function and pharmacological response to drugs (Kennedy 1980, 475). This consideration is repeatedly reinforced by empirical demonstrations of interorganismic similarity in basic processes. For example, according to Donald Kennedy, former director of the FDA, of the eighteen agents known (in 1980) to cause cancer in human beings, all but two also cause cancer in animals. Similarly, in their review of the value of animal teratogenicity testing for predicting human risk, Brown and Fabro conclude that "virtually all chemicals thought to cause human birth defects also induce embryotoxicity in at least one laboratory animal species" (1983, 470). (Nevertheless, it also is true, as Brown and Fabro point out, that interspecies comparisons often show qualitative differences in types of teratogenic effects as well as quantitative differences in dose-response relationships [p. 470].)

One must also consider, in testimony to the generalizability of animal research, its often demonstrated applicability to the solution of many biomedical questions as well as medical problems afflicting human beings. In an issue highlighting the benefits of animal research, the *American Journal of Public Health* stressed the contributions—in other words, the generalizability—of animal research to the understanding of basic anatomical and physiological processes in man; to the understanding of nutrition, including metabolism and dietary essentials such as vitamins and minerals, and the understanding of nutritional problems, including the role of nutrition in the prevention and management of illness; to the development of advanced surgical techniques, including hemorrhagic shock, cardiac lesions, and organ transplantation; to the isolation of hormones; and to the development of drugs useful in the regulation of organ function and in chemotherapy for infectious, parasitic, allergic, inflammatory, and cardiovascular diseases (McCann and Stare 1967; Robinson 1967; Winterscheid 1967).

Most scientists hold that these biomedical milestones would
never have been reached without the animal research that preceded them.

In summary, all the evidence available suggests that it
would be a serious error in judgment not to admit data obtained on animals to the consideration of teratogenicity in
humans.

Dosage: The Bridge from Research to Real Life

Another question that may be raised about generalizability of
the experimental studies summarized in tables 14 and 15 is that
many have used doses exceeding those generally used in therapeutic or clinical situations. The major reason for using high
doses in these experimental studies is an economic one. The
smaller the dose, the larger the number of animals needed to
demonstrate adverse effects, if such exist, and the larger the
number of animals needed, the more prohibitive the cost of
research (Kennedy 1980).

If there is a high probability that the dose-response relationship for a particular drug is continuous and linear, then it is
valid to extrapolate from the large doses often used in experimental studies to the smaller doses characteristic of clinical
use. For some types of agents, e.g., certain carcinogens, linear
extrapolation to the low-dose range may be less paradigmatic
than a discontinuous nonlinear function characterized by a
"safe" threshold at the low-dose end (Williams and Weisburger 1983). A linear model may also be less appropriate in
considering structurally teratogenic effects, many of which are
qualitative or binary in nature, e.g., alive or dead (Wilson
1977, 60–62). However, behaviorally teratogenic effects are
for the most part continuously distributed events of a quantitative nature, e.g., a range of test scores. Under these conditions, linear extrapolation from high dose to low is warranted.
Furthermore, in the absence of certain knowledge about linearity, the *assumption* of linearity is the more conservative posi-

tion and thus the one to be given priority in the interests of promoting and maintaining public health.

Design: The Bridge from Real Life to Research

A different question may be raised about the scientific value of the methodology employed in the human studies summarized in tables 14 and 15 (chap. 4) as well as those reviewed in table 1 (chap. 1). That question concerns the fact that almost all studies assessing effects on humans of teratogens or suspected teratogens are observational in design rather than experimental. In an observational study, also known as a quasi-experimental or correlational study, the investigator simply records what happens or has happened to the subjects being observed. In an experimentally designed study, also known as a randomized control or interventional study, the investigator randomly assigns subjects to experimental and control groups, thereby maximizing the probability that the groups are equivalent in all respects save that imposed by the experimental treatment and also maximizing confidence in a cause/effect interpretation of the results.

In human research involving suspected teratogens, including drugs, ethical constraints usually dicatate the use of an observational design: Since the fetus rarely requires or desires drug therapy, the anticipated benefit to it (zero) would be less than the anticipated risk (greater than zero) imposed by using an experimental model. (However, investigators can sometimes take advantage of "experiments in nature" such as the effects on offspring of drugs administered during labor and delivery.)

Experimental studies are generally valued more than observational studies because of the greater probability that a cause-effect interpretation of results is valid. Nevertheless, the preferred status of experimental studies does not mean that conclusions drawn from observational studies are invalid. As the Surgeon General's Advisory Committee on Smoking and Health (*Smoking and Health* 1964) pointed out, after grappling with the same problem of design and interpretation, the confidence that must be accorded cause-effect conclusions drawn from observational studies increases in proportion to the extent that those studies meet the following conditions:

- The association (or correlation) under consideration has been replicated and is consistent.
- The association is strong and shows a dose/effect relationship.
- The association is specific.
- The alleged cause preceded the effect.
- A cause/effect interpretation is compatible with known facts about relevant biological processes under investigation and/or with known facts about the natural history and biology of the disease under investigation. (See also Erickson 1981.)

To illustrate the application of these points, consider the body of evidence showing an association between obstetrical medication and adverse neurobehavioral outcome in infants (reviewed in chap. 1 and summarized in table 1).

- The association has been replicated in forty-seven studies carried out by different investigators using different methods. A few of these studies, e.g., Kron, Stein, and Goddard (1966), were experimental in design; their results agree with those obtained in observational studies. It should also be noted that none of the studies reported contradictory findings, i.e., that obstetrical medication was associated with improved neurobehavioral functioning.
- The correlations between obstetrical medication and adverse neurobehavioral functioning found in these studies are relatively strong, considering their small sample sizes as well as the magnitudes of correlations usually found in research involving behavioral variables. Moreover, the

adverse effects of relatively heavy toxic burdens (e.g., general anesthetics) are greater than those associated with less heavy toxic burdens (e.g., local anesthetics).

• The associations are specific in the sense that those neurobehavioral functions most affected are served by structures which are the least developed at time of birth.

• A cause/effect interpretation is supported by temporal considerations. That is, obstetric drug administration always precedes the appearance of adverse effects and not vice versa.

• A cause/effect interpretation is compatible with known biological facts: Obstetrical drugs cross the placenta easily and quickly. They readily pass through incompletely developed blood/brain barriers. They concentrate in brain structures that are still developing and therefore at high risk to damage. These toxic agents cannot readily be transformed to nontoxic compounds since the liver enzyme systems are functionally immature, and they cannot readily be excreted since kidney function is still immature.

After applying their criteria to the observational evidence on smoking and cancer, the Surgeon General's Advisory Committee judged that smoking does indeed cause cancer. By applying the same criteria to the observational evidence on obstetrical medications (table 1, chap. 1) and other drugs implicated in the production of teratogenic effects (tables 14 and 15, chap. 4), one is obliged to conclude that such agents do cause adverse neurobehavioral effects in exposed infants.

Mothers' Information about Drugs

The greater the probability that a drug may have adverse fetal effects, the more important it is, from an ethical point of view, that women who are pregnant or at risk of becoming pregnant have full information about that drug in order to exercise competence in deciding whether or not to consume it, i.e., to base an informed decision on reflective assessment of benefits to oneself versus risks to one's baby. Complete information is also important from a legal point of view, since most of the drugs administered obstetrically have never been approved for that purpose and therefore require mother's written informed consent before their administration.

A major purpose of this study was to find out how much drug information mothers have when they make such decisions. The basic results may be summarized as follows.

- For drugs consumed prenatally, the mean information score for all three groups was only 2.04 out of a possible 9 points. Most mothers knew the drug names and their expected action. Yet fewer than 2 percent of Hospital Mothers, 5 percent of Center Mothers, and 10 percent of Home Mothers were aware of the drug's potential for adverse fetal effects (table 18, chap. 4).
- For drugs administered intrapartally, the mean information score was .29 for Hospital Mothers. Only 2 percent of these Mothers could name the drugs they received, and 96 percent were not aware they had received one or more drugs actually administered to them.
- Those mothers with the most drug exposure had the lowest drug information scores. The mean prenatal drug exposure score for Hospital Mothers was twice that for Home Mothers, whereas the information score for Hospital Mothers was half that for Home Mothers.

The possible reasons why mothers do not have adequate information about the drugs they consume or are administered will be explored before turning to a discussion of the correlates of drug information.

Why Are Mothers Uninformed?

There are several possible reasons why women don't have information about the drugs they consume. One is that they don't want the information. Physicians often advance this as a reason for not providing more drug information to their patients (Moris, Mazis, and Gordon 1977). The present data fail to support such an explanation. When respondents were asked at the conclusion of the interview whether they would like less drug information, the same amount of information, or more information in advance of a subsequent pregnancy, a majority indicated a preference for more information. Further, those respondents who had the least information about drugs (Hospital Mothers) were the most eager to have more information.

This preference for information and shared decision making accords with previous studies' consistent findings that the large majority of consumers want information on drugs and everything else affecting their health and well-being (Alfidi 1971; Boreham and Gibson 1978; Fleckenstein et al. 1976; Gotsch and Liguori 1982; Mazis, Morris, and Gordon 1978; Michael and Bordley 1982; Morris and Kanouse 1981; Morris, Mazis, and Gordon 1977; Ryan and McMahon 1977; Shapiro et al. 1983).

The desire for health-related information, formerly attributed to younger and better-educated people, is no longer confined to these groups. It is now manifested widely and equally across all age and educational segments of the population (President's Commission 1982, 6, 7). Some of the specific desires include the following:

- 95 percent of Americans want to be told everything about their condition and treatment, including risks and side effects, even when the balance of such news is unfavorable (Harris, Boyle, and Brounstein 1982; see also Alfidi 1971; Fleckenstein et al. 1976).
- 91 percent want to decide treatment alternatives—either as sole decision maker or through shared decision making—with their doctors (Harris, Boyle, and Brounstein 1982).
- American health consumers want frankness rather than reassurance (Morris and Kanouse 1981).

- They want their own medical records (Michael and Bordley 1982).
- 89 percent of the public feel that patient rights to such information should be protected by law (Harris, Boyle, and Brounstein 1982).
- 72 percent feel that a doctor should be held legally liable for failing to inform patients fully and completely about the risks associated with a medical procedure (Harris, Boyle, and Brounstein 1982).
- 92 percent want full-length, detailed, comprehensive patient package inserts (Mazis, Morris, and Gordon 1978).
- 66 percent feel that it is primarily the doctor's responsibility to make sure patients are fully informed about their conditions and treatments (Harris, Boyle, and Brounstein 1982).
- 44 percent believe that when patients don't understand their medical treatment, it is always or often because the doctor did not explain it well (Harris, Boyle, and Brounstein 1982).
- 38 percent would even be willing to pay more if their doctors would spend more time explaining things about their routine care (Harris, Boyle, and Brounstein 1982).
- 36 percent have changed doctors because of some disagreement involving information and/or decision making (Harris, Boyle, and Brounstein 1982).
- 51 percent have taken the initiative in seeking a second opinion from another doctor (Harris, Boyle, and Brounstein 1982).

All of this suggests that our respondents were uninformed about drugs for other reasons than a lack of desire for information about those drugs.

A second possible explanation for women not having drug information is that although physicians may have given the information to their female patients, the women were intellectually incapable of understanding it. According to the findings of the President's Commission, 56 percent of the physicians interviewed cite their estimate of the patient's ability to understand the treatment or condition as the primary factor influencing the extent of information disclosure (Harris, Boyle, and Brounstein 1982, 121). One doctor summed it up by saying that women are unreliable and that physicians are solely competent to understand or provide medical information and as a consequence, solely capable of making decisions (Sweeney and Stern 1973). According to another physician, "You just can't give women information without causing a lot of trouble" (Ruzek 1978, 113).

Physicians' opinions to the contrary, empirical data do not support the presumption that men are superior to women in intellectual ability. Even disparity in educational attainment is no barrier to understanding: health-related information can be effectively transmitted at the elementary grade levels. The argument that women are incapable of assimilating information is not defensible.

Nevertheless, the point should also be made that most patients feel intimidated by physicians and fail to ask questions because they fear they will appear stupid (Rosenberg 1971) or their questions will appear "silly" (Ley and Spelman 1967).

Another possible reason why women lack information about drugs they consume is that they once had the information but forgot it. Memory fades with time, and nine months is a long time. Nevertheless, data from the present study suggest that forgetting is not a major explanation for lack of information: the mean information score for prenatal drugs, consumed up to nine months prior to the interview, was five times as high as the mean information score for the obstetric drugs to which these women were exposed only thirty-six hours before the interview. A number of studies have shown that the length of time elapsing between the presentation of information and the request for recall of that information is not significantly related to the amount of information remembered (Joyce et al. 1969; Ley and Spelman 1967; Ley et al. 1973; Ley et al. 1976).

Having concluded that women want information about the drugs they consume, that they are capable of assimilating such information, and that they have not forgotten the information they might once have had, we are left with the explanation that our subjects never received the information in the first place.

This inference is supported by the data on sources of information about prenatal drugs consumed by the respondents in this study. Our 602 mothers reported consuming a grand total of 2,077 drugs during their pregnancies (see table 20 in chap. 4, "Total Citations"). However, only 572 of the 2,077 drug intakes (28 percent) were accompanied by information provided by physicians. (Data on sources of information about drugs administered intrapartally could not be obtained because intrapartal drug information scores themselves were so insubstantial.)

The conclusion that our respondents never received drug information is also supported by mothers' responses to the general question, "Did your doctor discuss medications with you?" The majority of mothers in all groups reported that their doctors had never discussed medications with them (see table 23, chap. 4).

Data from other studies also support the conclusion that physicians do not provide their patients with information about drugs or other medical procedures (Boreham and Gibson 1978; Gray 1975; Harris, Boyle, and Brounstein 1982; Kirke 1980; Korsch and Negrete 1972; Lidz and Meisel 1982; Morris, Mazis, and Gordon 1977; Schultz, Pardee, and Ensinck 1975; Svarsted and Lipton 1977; Waitzkin and Stoeckle 1976). For example, and as noted earlier, Harris, Boyle, and Brounstein (1982) found that 94 percent of the public want their doctor to tell them everything, no matter how unfavorable. Yet the same investigators found that less than one in ten doctors (9 percent) actually do tell their patients everything about their conditions or treatments (p. 123). From their observational study of informed consent, described above, Lidz and Meisel (1982) flatly concluded that " 'Disclosure' does not typically occur" and that informed " 'consent' does not exist" (p. 401). This is true even when the medical procedure is experimental, and informed consent is required by law (Gray 1975; Schultz, Pardee, and Ensinck 1975). Furthermore, physicians are particularly prone to nondisclosure when they deal with female patients (Armitage, Schneiderman, and Bass 1979; Danziger 1978), black patients (Gray 1975), and clinic patients or those of lower socioeconomic status (Gray 1975; Shapiro et al. 1983).

Why Don't Physicians Provide Information?

Having established physicians' failure to provide drug information as the chief reason for women not having it, the next question to address is why physicians don't provide their patients with information about this important aspect of their health care.

In a report written for the President's Commission on Ethical Problems, Kaufmann (1982) suggests that one reason is economic. Informing takes time, and, for the professional, time is money. As Kaufmann notes, a hands-on physical examination is a billable charge, but a doctor-patient conversation is not. One of our subjects recounted trying to discuss some personal medical issues with her doctor. "He got more and more nervous and finally blurted out, 'But I have no way to bill you for all this talk!' That was the last question I ever asked him."

Still, the argument that economics silences information is a superficial one that does not bear up to scrutiny. Information can be provided in a variety of ways. Its presentation is not limited to one-on-one interpersonal interactions. Information can be effectively and economically conveyed by one person's talking to a large audience. It can also be conveyed by impersonal modes of presentation, including books, printed articles, computer programs, television, and films. Further, in a personal presentation, the presenter does not have to be a doctor. Nurses, pharmacists, physician assistants, and other health professionals are amply qualified to convey information about drugs to patients and other consumers. However, doctors choose not to use cost-effective modes of communication or to relinquish their function as informational gatekeeper to other health professionals. As Ehrenreich and Ehrenreich have observed, "What is especially significant is that the doctors have held on to their monopoly over communication with patients: nurses, technicians, and others may chat, but they cannot comment on your X-rays, or reveal so much as your temperature" (1974, 31).

All in all, one must conclude that physicians' failure to inform patients or to allow others to do so is a matter of motivation rather than economics—at least not economic in the direct or immediate sense that Kaufmann meant.

Information and Medical Power

If the cost of providing information is not the prime reason for its scarcity, what is? Many have suggested that power is the culprit. "Medical knowledge is seen as part of the professional property of the physician. Sharing information with patients may be construed as undercutting the status and authority of the physician in the treatment relationship" (Kaufmann 1982, App. I: 140). And according to Waitzkin and Waterman (1976), "There appears little reason for this low level of communication, other than the preservation of the physicans' dominant position in the doctor-patient relationship. To the extent that doctors try to narrow the competence gap by offering detailed explanations of illness and therapy, they also give up the power which depends on patients' ignorance" (p. 14).

Lukes (1974) has analyzed general theoretical views of power in terms of their "dimensionality." According to the one-dimensional view, the defining conditions are basically two parties, A and B, each of whom has an interest different from the other's and each of whom is consciously aware of those interests as well as the existence of a conflict between

them. The presence and locus of power is determined by see-
ing whose interest prevails as the outcome of pitting those
interests against each other in a decision-making encounter.
This has been called by others "outcome control." (See review
by Seligman and Miller 1979.) The overt conflict characterizing one-dimensional power does not often occur in doctor/
patient relationships.

In the two-dimensional view of power, both parties are also
aware of their own interests, but A manipulates the situation
so as to exclude B's conflicting interest(s) from entering the
decision-making arena. Others have called this "agenda control" (Seligman and Miller 1979) and "topical autonomy"
(Danziger 1978). As Danziger has noted, "In the encounter
with the patient, a physician has the prerogative to define what
is therapeutic and what is outside the bounds of consideration,
what aspects of the case shall be deemed relevant and irrelevant, and what topics are open and what topics are not open
for discussion between doctor and patient" (p. 360).

The two-dimensional view suggests that women may not obtain information because the obstetrician shapes the interaction
so that the patient's concerns are not discussed. Indeed, agenda
control appeared to be a major operative force in a recent study
by Shapiro et al. (1983). In that study, women were given a
questionnaire at their initial obstetrical visit and the same questionnaire at about thirty-six weeks. On the first questionnaire,
clients were asked to indicate whether they would like to obtain
information from their doctors on each of the listed topics. The
second questionnaire requested that clients indicate which topics were discussed with their obstetrician and whether further
discussion was desired. Results showed that the women never
had had the opportunity to discuss with their obstetricians most
of the topics about which they had initially wanted information.

The three-dimensional level represents the most subtle form
of power. In this scenario, party A manipulates the situation
so that party B is not aware that a conflict of interests exists
and therefore is not aware of the opportunity or need to pro-

tect his or her own interest in the decisions affecting it. Indeed, B may not even be aware that such decisions are being made. As Lukes describes this form of power, "it [is] the supreme and most insidious exercise of power to prevent people, to whatever degree, from having grievances by shaping their perceptions, cognitions and preferences in such a way that they accept their role in the existing order of things, either because they can see or imagine no alternative to it. . .or because they value it as divinely ordained and beneficial" (1974, 24).

The key to three-dimensional power is informational ownership or, more precisely, informational disparity: A is gatekeeper to information affecting B's interests; A has the information and B doesn't. Further, B isn't aware s(he) needs the information or perhaps that the information even exists.

This three-dimensional conception of power is the one most characteristic not just of obstetrics but the whole of American medicine, according to Starr (1982). Starr's social history of this professional group starts from the fact that American medicine was for centuries "a relatively weak, traditional profession of minor economic consequence" (p. 4). Within the last century, however, it has risen to a position of sovereignty unparalleled among other professional groups in the United States and has been able to turn its authority into "social privilege, economic power, and political influence" (p. 5). How did this come about?

According to Starr, the medical profession's power has its origins in dependence on medical authority.[13] The dependence

---

13. Starr also cites what he terms the "legitimation" of the medical profession as an important contributor to its meteoric rise to power. "The legitimation of professional authority involves three distinctive claims: first, that the knowledge and competence of the profesional have been validated by a community of his or her peers; second, that this consensually validated knowledge and competence rest on rational scientific grounds; and third, that the professional's judgment and advice are oriented toward a set of substantive values, such as health" (1982, 15). The mechanics supporting legitimation are, in Starr's opinion, standardized education and licensing.

of Americans on their physicians, according to Starr, rested initially and primarily on informational disparity between patient and physician—a disparity that took a quantum leap with the revolutionary growth in the twentieth century of specialized medical knowledge and technology. Yet, as one physician has pointed out (Mendelsohn 1979), any patient with a sixth-grade education and a medical dictionary can span this informational gap. To guard against such a possibility, the medical profession has reinforced the dependency by institutionalizing it, i.e., by successfully promulgating laws and regulations restricting medical education, licensing, and the right to practice "medicine"; restricting access to drugs and therapeutic devices; restricting the use and control of hospitals; controlling certification of patients (e.g., life insurance, health insurance, sick leave); controlling third party payments to health professionals and health institutions; and controlling the funding available for medical research.

The medical profession has also reinforced public dependence in ways that are basically semantic rather than legal or regulatory. One important instance of this is medicine's creation of a technical jargon that functions as an informational barrier to those outside medical ranks. A pertinent example is the FDA's regulation requiring manufacturers of prescription drugs to use language on drug labels that is "unintelligible to the layman" (U.S. Food and Drug Administration 1938). In connection with this, note that the coded language of prescriptions themselves also renders these directions to pharmacists unintelligible to consumers. As one scientist remarked, "the use of jargon rather than non-technical terms in the interaction [between doctor and patient] maintains the esoteric nature of scientific knowledge, inaccessible to the layperson. . .[and] mystification, either through information control or use of jargon, maintains stratification within the relationship" (Waitzkin 1979, 606, 607). Some humorists have suggested that a medical degree is not just a certification of curative skills but a certification of linguistic skills as well.

A second important way in which the medical profession has used language to increase public dependence is by expanding the definitional limits of what is commonly or legally regarded as medicine's exclusive territory. For example, alcoholism was once regarded as a moral problem to be handled by persons of the cloth and officers of the law. Through the efforts of the medical profession, alcoholism is now labeled "a disease" and thus, by extension, a province of the medical empire. Similarly, childbirth, once regarded as a natural physiological function requiring the assistance of female relatives, friends, and mid-wives, has now been successfully reclassified as "a disease," or at best a high-risk state, requiring hospitalization, a host of technological interventions, and medical supervision.

Finally, with respect to power, it should be noted that the general problem of disparity in power between doctor and patient is exacerbated in the particular case of obstetrics by an additional disparity in gender: all the patients are women and almost all the doctors are men. The relationship of gender to social influence has been repeatedly documented in the social science research literature as well as the feminist literature— see, for example, the scholarly review by Eagly (1983) and the feminist exhortations by Ehrenreich and English (1973) and Frankfort (1972). Following Eagly's analysis, the situation may be summarized as follows.

- Societal norms confer legitimacy on the authority of persons occupying high positions in any hierarchy, so that "the individual higher in the hierarchy is believed to have the right to exert influence by virtue of his or her position in the social system, and the individual lower in the hierarchy is believed to have the obligation to comply with the demands that are made" (Eagly 1983, 971).
- Normative influences are very effective. Persons vested with authority obtain ready compliance with their requests, as demonstrated repeatedly by social psychologists for a variety of contexts (e.g., Milgram 1965, 1974).

- There are large sex differences within almost all functioning hierarchies in our society. "Given the legitimate authority inherent in higher status positions, men . . . have
greater power to influence others and to resist being influ-
enced merely as a product of their greater concentration
in higher status positions" (Eagly 1983, 972).

Considering this compounded power differential from a historical point of view, it is hardly surprising that male physicians
targeted female patients and midwives early on nor is it surprising that they were so successful in their appropriation of midwifery. According to historian Paul Starr (1982), the shift from
midwives to physicians began over two hundred years ago in the
United States when, in 1763, the first male physician took up
obstetric practice. By 1815, the Philadelphia city directory listed
twenty-one women and twenty-three men as practicing midwives; in 1819 it listed thirteen women and forty-two men; by
1824, only six female midwives remained in Philadelphia's official roster (Starr 1982, 49–50). Starr goes on to point out, "No
licensing laws compelled the shift, and though physicians had
economic motives to take over midwifery, they were in no position to force women to accept them. . . .[the] probable explanation is that well-to-do women had come to accept the physicians'
claims of superior skill" (p. 50).

Medical Power and the FDA

The assumption underlying the foregoing discussion is that
physicians, as the fiduciaries and major providers of health
care during pregnancy and childbirth, also bear primary responsibility for providing information to their patients about
health care during pregnancy, including information about
drugs. Nevertheless, at the institutional level there is another
storehouse of information and another set of gatekeepers who
have taken authority with respect to drugs and consumers and
are thereby accountable to the public.

In June, 1938, Congress passed legislation creating the Food and Drug Administration. One of the two major purposes of this legislation was to protect American consumers from missing and misleading information about drugs as well as other products.[14] Congressional intent was not to restrict drug sales nor to restrict self-medication but rather to aid consumers in obtaining full and accurate information about drugs and other products (Temin 1980, 54). Six months later, however, the FDA reversed congressional intent when it issued general regulations translating the abstract language of the enabling legislation into the FDA's own concrete ground rules of operational procedure (U.S. Food and Drug Administration 1938). The importance of these regulations with respect to drugs was that they divided drugs into two classes (prescription and nonprescription), prohibited the direct sale of prescription drugs to consumers, and also effectively prohibited the dissemination of information about prescription drugs to consumers. The FDA closed the gate on drug information by decreeing that all labeling for prescription products "appear only in such medical terms as are not likely to be understood by the ordinary individual" (U.S. Food and Drug Administration 1938). As Temin (1980) notes in his historical account of the FDA, "Drug manufacturers and the FDA would now decide which drugs consumers could select from: consumers were no longer considered capable of selecting drugs on their own. The government had delegated the consumer's choice to manufacturers and doctors" (p. 54). Temin goes on to note, "One effect of this change in underlying assumptions [from the Congressional assumption of a competent consumer to the FDA assumption of an incompetent one] was to benefit doctors. By curbing self-medication, the government channeled business to the

---

14. Public Law No. 717, 75th Cong., Chap. 675, 3d Sess. S. 5. An act to prohibit the movement in interstate commerce of adulterated and misbranded food, drugs, devices, and cosmetics, and for other purposes. (The short title is "Federal Food, Drug, and Cosmetic Act.") Note the title's emphasis on the provision of accurate information ("misbranded" food, etc.).

doctors and increased the value of their licenses" (p. 55). In effect, "The government had appointed doctors as the consumers' purchasing agents" (p. 47).[15]

During the almost half century of its existence, the FDA's policy of withholding drug information from consumers, eliminating consumer choice, and increasing consumer dependence on the medical profession has continued with unwavering consistency. The most recent example of note was cancellation of the program to provide consumers with the drug information contained in patient package inserts. In fact, so effective is this policy that most consumers have less than accurate information about the FDA itself or about the way in which the FDA actually functions in the regulation of drugs and drug information.

In support of this conclusion, we present the results of informal research carried out to ascertain how much accurate information consumers have about the ways in which the FDA chooses to regulate drugs for the protection of consumer interests. The ten-item test shown in table 24 was devised for this purpose. The first three items focus on general information about drugs; the remaining seven items bear on the FDA's regulating authority and mode of functioning. The test was administered to eleven couples in childbirth education classes who had received two hours of instruction on obstetrical drugs, sixty-two pharmacy students who had successfully completed a course in pharmacology and were in their last year of professional training, and one practicing obstetrician.

The results show that even these relatively sophisticated individuals, who have some information about drugs in general (items 1–3), have relatively little information about the FDA's drug-regulating functions (items 4–10). These results suggest that the FDA, in addition to withholding from the public information about drugs, also sequesters information about its regulating functions with respect to drugs.

---

15. For an unabridged history of the birth of the FDA, see *A Legislative History of the Federal Food, Drug, and Cosmetic Act and Its Amendments.* Washington, D.C.: General Printing Office, 1979. Vols. 1–24.

TABLE 24. Percentage of Correct Answers on a Test of Information about Drugs and the FDA

Test Item	Childbirth Education Participants ($N = 22$)	Graduating Pharmacy Students ($N = 62$)	Obstetrician ($N = 1$)
1. Nonprescription products sold over-the-counter are not "real drugs."	100	100	100
2. If a drug is safe for adults, it's safe for children in smaller amounts.	100	100	100
3. The number of obstetric drugs administered is decreasing.	27	40	100
Average, Items 1-3	76	80	100
4. By congressional mandate, the FDA is responsible for approving drugs on the grounds of safety and efficacy before those drugs are marketed or released for clinical use. Therefore, a marketed drug is both safe and effective.	82	61	100
5. Testing for teratogenicity is required by law or by rules and regulations that have the force of law.	55	48	0

6. Drugs are tested for both structural and behavioral teratogenicity prior to their approval.	55	68	0
7. Testing of a drug for safety and efficacy is carried out by FDA or by an independent laboratory under FDA supervision.	18	61	0
8. By congressional mandate, the FDA can approve for marketing or release only those drugs scientifically proven to be safe and effective.	59	34	100
9. Consumers and researchers may examine pre-marketing adverse drug reaction data after a drug has been approved for marketing and clinical use.	18	23	0
10. After a drug is marketed, FDA systematically surveys for adverse drug reactions that may not have been spotted in the small sample, premarketing research.	50	71	100
Average, Items 4–10	52	48	43

Note: Correct answers are all false. Thanks to Dr. Robert S. K. Young, FDA, for his help in constructing this test.

125

Correlates of Maternal Information about Drugs

Having established that most mothers have little information about their prenatal medications and even less about their intrapartal medications, we then explored the possible reasons why mothers are so poorly informed. The final question concerns those variables that were associated with maternal information about drugs.

Variables correlating significantly with Hospital Mothers' information about prenatally consumed drugs included age, education, race, intrapartal drug information, locus of control scores, and health-promoting behavior scores. In all cases, significance levels were less than .0001. Thus, a profile of the Hospital Mother with the most information about the drugs she consumed while pregnant reveals someone who is older, better educated, white, has more information about the obstetric drugs she received, views her own decisions and actions as effective forces in shaping her life, and engages in more behaviors known to promote wellness and prevent health problems. The last two variables represent the extent to which the individual perceives and acts in ways consonant with controlling the environment rather than being controlled by it. The results for these two variables are consistent with earlier research showing that individuals with relatively high internal locus of control scores have high information scores (e.g., Lefcourt 1976), use information effectively (e.g., Prociuk and Breen 1977), are attentive to information (e.g., Lefcourt and Wine 1969), and have good memory for important information (e.g., Phares 1968).

Variables significantly associated with Hospital Mothers' information about intrapartally administered drugs include education, race, prenatal drug information, and information about drugs in general. The profile of an informed Hospital Mother reveals a person who is better educated, white, has more information about the drugs she consumed while pregnant, and more information about drugs in general. Note, however, that information about intrapartal drug administration was not related to either locus of control or engagement in health-promoting behaviors (in contrast to the highly significant associations between these variables and prenatal drug information). Note also that there was no relationship between the number of drugs Hospital Mothers chose to consume prenatally and the number administered to them intrapartally by medical personnel. Both sets of facts confirm earlier findings (Brown, Manning, and Grodin 1972) that women forfeit decision-making control when they choose to deliver in-hospital. As McManus et al. (1982) observed, "an internal locus of control and a belief in one's own decision-making abilities are irrelevant or even inappropriate in the hospital setting because control is directly in the hands of more powerful others" (p. 28).

Summary

This study investigated prenatal and intrapartal use of drugs, the status of those drugs with respect to safety for the fetus or neonate; and the amount of information mothers have about the drugs they have consumed or that have been administered to them.

We found that mothers delivering in-hospital or at a freestanding birth center consumed more drugs during their pregnancies than mothers choosing to deliver at home. During childbirth, Hospital Mothers were also the recipients of more drugs than Center or Home Mothers. For most of these drugs, teratogenicity has either never been assessed or is implicated by the research literature.

Apropos of drug information, the data indicated that mothers knew very little about the drugs they consume during pregnancy and even less about the drugs administered to them during childbirth. Home Mothers were significantly better informed than Center Mothers who, in turn, were significantly better informed than Hospital Mothers.

After exploring possible reasons for the paucity of drug

128   Medication in Maternity

information, the most likely explanation appeared to be that, in the interests of maintaining a position of power, physicians simply do not provide information, even though ethical and legal considerations oblige them to do so. At the institutional level, the FDA pursues a similar policy of nondisclosure with respect to both drug information and its own operations.

Suggestions for Future Research

Medical personnel are not the only sources of information about drugs, and pregnancy is not the only period for seeking out such information. Information about drugs—and information on how to get information—can be incorporated into high school health and science curricula during prepregnancy years. First of all, students could be taught some basic information about drugs and pregnancy. This might include what is currently known about the effects of commonly used medications, cigarettes, and alcohol on the unborn child. The incorporation of this information into the high school curricula would provide students with a solid introduction to the area as well as illustrate to them the importance of having information about the drugs they consume and thus motivate them to seek out such information in the future. Instruction about where to obtain such information and opportunities to practice obtaining it should also be included in the curricula so that students could develop information-seeking skills using such sources of information as pharmacists, libraries, and computer search facilities.

The variable most closely associated with differential drug intake and drug information was choice of birthplace. To a considerable extent, the same set of motives (independence? skepticism? desire for control?) that impels a woman to reject the hospital as a preferred place of birth must also be operative when she rejects drugs as the therapy of first choice. One means of examining the motivations underlying these decisions would be to systematically investigate womens' reasons for choosing between traditional and nontraditional places of birth. An understanding of these reasons would provide valuable insight into the differences between women choosing the various alternatives as well as provide information about the positive and negative aspects of those decisions. Cognitive, perceptual, and personality measures could be used to assess those factors contributing to decision making. A variety of measures would be useful in uncovering individual differences in this regard including assessments of independence versus dependence, perceived locus of control, trust versus distrust in others, acceptance versus rejection of authoritarian attitudes, and pursuit versus avoidance of information as a general cognitive style.

A final suggestion for future research concerns not just the substantive issues with which it might be concerned, but the breadth and scope of investigations. Specifically, we refer to the need for interdisciplinary studies that are focused on primary causes of learning disorders, that are follow-up if not longitudinal in design, and that include educators among the research designers of the dependent variables. The new disciplines of behavioral teratology and developmental toxicology have amassed considerable evidence demonstrating the immediate behavioral effects of chemical insult to the developing central nervous system. Nevertheless, long-term investigations, using longitudinal or follow-up designs and dependent measures of maximal ecological validity, are practically nonexistent. Such studies, involving extensive assessment of educational achievements and educational problems, including learning disorders and their antecedents, are sorely needed.

Appendixes

Health-Promoting Behavior Items

Did you use (during pregnancy):

Coffee per day	No = 1	1–2 = 2	3–4 = 3	5–6 = 4	> 6 = 5
	caffeinated = 1	decaffeinated = 2			
Tea per day	No = 1	1–2 = 2	3–4 = 3	5–6 = 4	> 6 = 5
"Coke" per day	No = 1	1–4 = 2	5–8 = 3	9–12 = 4	> 12 = 5
Cigarettes per day	No = 1	1–6 = 2	7–13 = 3	14–20 = 4	> 20 = 5

_____ Brand _____ mg tar

By the way, do you smoke in bed?
No = 1   occasionally = 3   yes = 5

Beer per day	No = 1	1/week = 2	2–6/week = 3	1/day = 4	>1/day = 5
Wine per day	No = 1	1/week = 2	2–6/week = 3	1/day = 4	> 1/day = 5
Mixed drinks	No = 1	1/week = 2	2–6/week = 3	1/day = 4	> 1/day = 5
Marijuana per day	No = 1	1/week = 2	2–6/week = 3	1/day = 4	> 1/day = 5
Other social drugs	No = 1	1/week = 2	2–6/week = 3	1/day = 4	> 1/day = 5

Do you participate in any physical activities, e.g., jogging, swimming? How often?

1 = _____ daily
2 = _____ 2/week
3 = _____ 1/week
4 = _____ every other week
5 = _____ No

Do you participate in a vigorous exercise program? How often?

1 = _____ daily
2 = _____ 2/week
3 = _____ 1/week

4 = _____ every other week
5 = _____ No

How much did you weigh before your pregnancy?_____

How tall are you?

1 = _____	< 5′	8 = _____	5′7′′
2 = _____	5′1′′	9 = _____	5′8′′
3 = _____	5′2′′	10 = _____	5′9′′
4 = _____	5′3′′	11 = _____	5′10′′
5 = _____	5′4′′	12 = _____	5′11′′
6 = _____	5′5′′	13 = _____	6′
7 = _____	5′6′′	14 = _____	> 6′

How often do you eat meat, fish, poultry, eggs or some other source of protein?

0 = _____ not codeable
1 = _____ 1/day
2 = _____ 2/week
3 = _____ 1/week
4 = _____ less often
5 = _____ never

How often do you eat fruit?

0 = _____ not codeable
1 = _____ 1/day
2 = _____ 2/week
3 = _____ 1/week
4 = _____ less often
5 = _____ never

How often do you eat vegetables?

0 = _____ not codeable
1 = _____ 1/day
2 = _____ 2/week
3 = _____ 1/week
4 = _____ less often
5 = _____ never

Do you examine your own breasts? How often?

1 = _____ 1/month

2 = _____ every other month
3 = _____ 2/year
4 = _____ 1/year
5 = _____ never

Do you get a PAP test routinely?
     No = 5   Yes = 1

Do you use dental floss? How often?
     1 = _____ 1/day
     2 = _____ sometimes
     3 = _____ never

Do you wear a seat belt or harness when you're in a car? How often?
     1 = _____ always
     2 = _____ most of the time
     3 = _____ sometimes
     4 = _____ rarely
     5 = _____ never

How many hours a day do you watch T.V.?
     1 = _____ none
     2 = _____ 2 hours
     3 = _____ 3 hours
     4 = _____ 4 hours
     5 = _____ > 4 hours

Have you ever taken a first aid course or are you familiar with first
aid procedures?
     No = 3   Yes = 1

Do you shop regularly at a health food store?
     No = 3   Yes = 1

Maternal Drug Consumption: Drug Ingredients and Products Containing Those Ingredients

Drug Ingredient	Drug Products
acetaminophen	CoTylenol, Comtrex, Datril, Excedrin, Excedrin PM, Nyquil, Percogesic, Sinutab, Tylenol, Tylenol #3, Tylenol with Codeine
acetic acid	Aci-Jel Therapeutic Vaginal Jelly
alginic acid	Gaviscon
allantoin	AVC Cream, Tegrin, Vagitrol
alphaprodine hydrochloride	Nisentil
aluminum glycinate	Bufferin
aluminum hydroxide	Di-Gel, Dristan, Gaviscon, Gelusil, Maalox, Mylanta
aminocrine hydrochloride	AVC Cream, Vagitrol
aminophylline	aminophylline
ampicillin	ampicillin
anise	Black Draught
antazoline phosphate	Vasacon-A
aspirin	Alka-Seltzer, Alka-Seltzer Plus, Anacin, aspirin, BC Powder, Bufferin, Coricidin-D, Dristan, Excedrin, Sine-Off
atropine sulfate	atropine sulfate, Lomotil
beechwood	Creomulsion
benzalkonium chloride	Neo-Synephrine, Privine Nose Drops
benzocaine	Anbesol, Bicozene Cream, Vagisil

Drug Ingredient	Drug Products
bismuth subsalicylate	Pepto-Bismol
boric acid	Aci-Jel Therapeutic Vaginal Jelly, Vasocon-A
bupivacaine hydrochloride	Marcaine
butorphanol tartrate	Stadol
caffeine	Anacin, BC Powder, Dristan, Excedrin
calcium carbonate	Chooz, Dicarbosil, Pepto-Bismol, Tums
camphor	Va-Tro-Nol, Vicks VapoRub
casanthranol	Pericolace
cascara	Creomulsion
cedar leaf oil	Vicks VapoRub
cephalexin	Keflex
cephradine	Velosef
cetearyl octonate	Pristeen
cetylpyridinium chloride	Massengill Disposable Douche
chlordiazepoxide hydrochloride	Librium
chlorobutanol	Asthma Nephrin
chloroprocaine hydrochloride	Nesacaine
chlorpheniramine maleate	Alka-Seltzer Plus, Allerphen, Chlor-Trimeton, CoTylenol, Comtrex, Contac, Coricidin-D, Novahistine, Sine-Offim* 230,390/
cholesterols	Phiso-Derm
cinnamon	Black Draught
citric acid	Alka-Seltzer, Phenergan Expectorant with Codeine, Summer's Eve
clindamycin hydrochloride	Cleocin
clomiphene citrate	Clomid
clove	Black Draught
coal tar extract	Tegrin
cod liver oil	Desitin
codeine phosphate	codeine phosphate, Phenergan Expectorant with Codeine, Tylenol #3, Tylenol with Codeine
codeine sulfate	codeine sulfate
cortisone acetate	cortisone acetate

Drug Ingredient	Drug Products
creosote	Creomulsion
cyclobenzaprine	Flexeril
dexamethasone	Decadron
dextromethorphan	Comtrex, Robistussin DM, Vicks Formula 44
dextrose	dextrose 5%/.2% sodium chloride solution
diazepam	Valium
digoxin	digoxin
dihydroxyaluminum sodium carbonate	Rolaids
dimenhydrinate	Dramamine
dioctyl sodium sulfosuccinate	Colace, Correctol, Pericolace
diphenhydramine hydrochloride	Benadryl
diphenoxylate	Lomotil
doxylamine succinate	Benedectin, Nyquil, Vicks Formula 44
entsufon sodium	Phiso-Derm
ephedrine sulfate	Chlor-Trimeton, ephedrine sulfate, Nyquil, Va-Tro-Nol
epinephrine hydrochloride	Asthma Nefrin, epinephrine hydrochloride, Primatene Mist
erythromycin	erythromycin
eucalyptol (eucalyptus oil)	Halls Mentholyptus Cough Drops, Listerine Lozenges, Va-Tro-Nol, Vicks VapoRub
fentanyl	Sublimaze
furosemide	Lasix
gentamicin	Garamycin
glycerin	Aci-Jel Therapeutic Vaginal Jelly, Anbesol
glycine	Afrin
gramicidin	Mycolog
guaifenesin	Robitussin, Robitussin DM
halothane	halothane
heparin sodium	heparin sodium
hexylresorcinol	Listerine Lozenges
hydralazine hydrochloride	Apresoline
hydroxyzine hydrochloride	Vistaril
insulin	insulin
iodine	Anbesol

Drug Ingredient	Drug Products
ipecac	Creomulsion, Phenergan Expectorant with Codeine
isopropanol myristate	FDS, Pristeen
isoxsuprine hydrochloride	Vasodilan
kaolin	Kaopectate, Parapectolin
ketamine hydrochloride	ketamine hydrochloride
lactic acid	Massengill Disposable Douche
lanolin	Desitin, FDS, Phiso-Derm
lidocaine hydrochloride	lidocaine hydrochloride, Xylocaine
live yeast extract	Preparation H
magaldrate	Riopan
magnesium carbonate	Bufferin, Dristan
magnesium hydroxide	Gelusil, Haley's M-O, Maalox, Milk of Magnesia, Mylanta
magnesium oxide	Di-Gel, Milk of Magnesia
magnesium sulfate	magnesium sulfate
magnesium trisilicate	Chooz, Gaviscon
menthol	Creomulsion, Halls Mentholyptus Cough Drops, Listerine Lozenges, Va-Tro-Nol, Vicks VapoRub
meperidine hydrochloride	Demerol
metaproterenol sulfate	Alupent, Metaprel
methenamine hippurate	Hiprex
methoxyflurane	Penthrane
methyl salicylate	Va-Tro-Nol
methylbenzethonium chloride	Norforms
methylene chloride	FDS
methylprednisolone	Medrol
methylprednisolone sodium succinate	Solu-Medrol
metronidazole	Flagyl
miconazole	Monistat
mineral oil	FDS, Haley's M-O
morphine sulfate	morphine sulfate
myristica oil	Vicks VapoRub
naloxone hydrochloride	Narcan
naphazoline hydrochloride	Privine Nose Drops, Vasocon-A
neomycin sulfate	Mycolog
nitrous oxide	nitrous oxide
nystatin	Mycolog, Mycostatin

Drug Ingredient	Drug Products
octoxynol	Massengill Disposable Douche
oxtriphylline	Choledyl
oxymetazoline hydrochloride	Afrin
oxyquinoline sulfate	Aci-Jel Therapeutic Vaginal Jelly
oxytocin	oxytocin, Pitocin
pancuronium bromide	Pavulon
paregoric	Parapectolin
pectin	Kaopectate, Parapectolin
penicillin	penicillin
pentobarbital	Nembutal
peppermint	Black Draught
peppermint oil	Dicarbosil, Milk of Magnesia, Tums
petrolatum	Desitin, Phiso-Derm
phenidamine tartrate	Dristan
pheniramine maleate	Triaminic Syrup
phenobarbital	phenobarbital
phenol	Anbesol, Chloraseptic Throat Spray
phenylephrine hydrochloride	CoTylenol, Dristan, Neo-Synephrine
phenylmercuric acetate	Vasocon-A
phenylmercuric nitrate	Preparation H
phenylpropanolamine hydrochloride	Comtrex, Contac, Coricidin-D, Novahistine, Sine-Off, Sinutab, Triaminic Syrup
phenyltoloxamine citrate	Percogesic, Sinutab
potassium chloride	BC Powder, potassium chloride
povidone-iodine	Betadine
prednisone	prednisone
procaine	Novacain
prochlorperazine	Compazine
progesterone	progesterone
promethazine hydrochloride	Phenergan, Phenergan Expectorant with Codeine
propoxyphene hydrochloride	Darvon
propoxyphene napsylate	Darvocet
propranolol hydrochloride	Inderal
pseudoephedrine hydrochloride	Actifed, Sudafed
psyllium mucilloid	Metamucil
pyridoxine hydrochloride	Bendectin

Drug Ingredient	Drug Products
pyrilamine maleate	Excedrin PM, Triaminic Syrup
resorcin	Bicozene Cream, Vagisil
ricinoleic acid	Aci-Jel Therapeutic Vaginal Jelly
ritodrine hydrochloride	ritodrine hydrochloride
salicylamide	BC Powder, Excedrin
secobarbital	secobarbital
senna	Black Draught, Fletcher's Castoria
shark liver oil	Preparation H
simethicone	Di-Gel, Gelusil, Mylanta
sodium bircarbonate	Alka-Seltzer, Gaviscon
sodium biphosphate	Fleet Enema
sodium carbonate	Vasocon-A
sodium chloride	Vasocon-A
sodium citrate	Phenergan Expectorant with Codeine, Summer's Eve
sodium hydroxide	Afrin
sodium phenolate	Chloraseptic Throat Spray
sodium phosphate	Fleet Enema
sodium thiopental	Pentothal
sorbitol	Afrin
succinylcholine chloride	Anectine
sulfabenzamide	Sultrin Triple Sulfa Cream
sulfacetamide	Sultrin Triple Sulfa Cream
sulfanilamide	AVC Cream, Vagitrol
sulfathiazole	Sultrin Triple Sulfa Cream
sulfisoxazole	Azogantrisin, Gantrisin
talc	Desitin
tetracaine hydrochloride	tetracaine hydrochloride
tetrahydrozaline	Visine
theophylline	Theo Dur
thymol	Vicks VapoRub
triamcinalone acetonide	Mycolog
triprolidine hydrochloride	Actifed
tubocurarine	curare
turpentine spirits	Vicks VapoRub
white pine	Creomulsion
wild cherry	Creomulsion
yellow phenolpthalein	Correctol, Ex-Lax, Feen-A-Mint
zinc oxide	Desitin
zinc sulfate	Summer's Eve

Numbered References for Tables 14 and 15

1. Gladstone, G. R.; Hordof, A.; and Gersony, W. M. 1975. "Propranolol Administration during Pregnancy: Effects on the Fetus." *Journal of Pediatrics* 86:962–64.

2. Gilbert, E. F., and Pistey, W. R. 1973. "Effect on the Offspring of Repeated Caffeine Administration to Pregnant Rats." *Journal of Reproduction and Fertility* 34:495–99.

3. Van Petten, G. R., and Willes, R. F. 1970. "β-Adrenoceptive Responses in the Unanaesthetized Ovine Foetus." *British Journal of Pharmacology* 38:572–82.

4. Warkany, J., and Takacs, E. 1959. "Experimental Production of Congenital Malformations in Rats by Salicylate Poisoning." *American Journal of Pathology* 35:315–31.

5. Corbett, T. H.; Cornell, R. G.; Endres, J. L.; and Millard, R. I. 1973. "Effects of Low Concentrations of Nitrous Oxide on Rat Pregnancy." *Anesthesiology* 39:299–301.

6. Hannah, R. S., and Moore, K. L. 1971. "Effects of Fasting and Insulin on Skeletal Development in Rats." *Teratology* 4:135–39.

7. Parabrook, G. D.; Mobbs, I.; and Mackenzie, J. 1965. "Effects of Nitrous Oxide on the Early Chick Embryo." *British Journal of Anaesthesia* 37:990–91.

8. Scaglione, S. 1962. "Osservazione e ricerche sull'azione dell'insulina sugli embrioni di ratte, gravide con microfotografie." *Acta Geneticae Medicae et Gemellologiae* 11:418–29.

9. Suzuki, M. R. 1970. "Effects of Oral Cyclofenil and Clomiphene, Ovulation Inducing Agents on Pregnancy and Fetuses in Rats." *Oyo Yakuri* 4:635–44.

10. Gordon, N. W.; Peer, L. A.; and Bernhard, W. G. 1961. "The Relation of the Teratogenic Action of Cortisone to Liver Transaminase Activity." *Biology of the Neonate* 3:36–48.

11. Arrington, L. R.; Taylor, R. N., Jr.; Ammerman, C. B.; and Shirley, R. L. 1965. "Effects of Excess Dietary Iodine upon Rabbits, Hamsters, Rats and Swine." *Journal of Nutrition* 87:394–98.

12. Fraser, F. C. 1969. "Gene-Environment Interactions in the Production of Cleft Palate." In *Methods for Teratological Studies in Animals and Man,* edited by H. Nishimura and J. R. Miller. Tokyo: Igaku Shoin.

13. Malakhovski, B. G., and Prozorovski, B. V. 1972. "Affection of the Brain of Rats which Sustained Intrauterine Action of Estrone and Progesterone." *Biulleten Eksperimentalnoi Biologii i Meditisiny* 74:34 (in Russian).

14. Goldstein, A., and Hazel, M. M. 1955. "Failure of an Antihistamine Drug to Prevent Pregnancy in the Mouse." *Endocrinology* 56:215–16.

15. Saxen, I. 1975. "Associations between Oral Clefts and Drugs Taken during Pregnancy." *International Journal of Epidemiology* 4:37–44.

16. Koeter, H. W. B. M., and Rodier, P. M. 1981. "Functional Development of Mice after Pre- or Postnatal Exposure to Inhalent Anesthetics." *Teratology* 24: 56A.

17. Hughes, J. G.; Ehemann, B.; and Brown, U. A. 1948. "Electroencephalography of the Newborn: III. Brain Potentials of Babies Born of Mothers Given 'Seconal Sodium.' " *American Journal of Diseases of Children* 76:626–33.

18. Robkin, M. A.; Shepard, T. H.; and Baum, D. 1974. "Autonomic Drug Effects on the Heart Rate of Early Rat Embryos." *Teratology* 9:35–44.

19. Dudley, A. W., Jr.; Chang, L. W.; and Katz, J. 1974. "Ultrastructural Evidence of Hepatic and Renal Changes in Neonatal Rats following in Uteral Exposure to Low Levels of Halothane." *Federation Proceedings* 33:625.

20. Pitel, M., and Lerman, S. 1964. "Further Studies on the Effects of Intrauterine Vasoconstrictors on the Fetal Rat Lens." *American Journal of Ophthalmology* 58:464–70.

21. Kron, R. E.; Stein, M.; and Goddard, K. E. 1966. "Newborn Sucking Behavior Affected by Obstetric Sedation." *Pediatrics* 37:1012–16.

22. McColl, J. D.; Robinson, S.; and Globus, M. 1967. "Effect of Some Therapeutic Agents on the Rabbit Fetus." *Toxicology and Applied Pharmacology* 10:244–52.

23. Drachman, D. B., and Coulombre, A. J. 1962. "Experimental Club Foot and Arthrogryposis Multiplex Congenita." *Lancet* 2:523–26.

24. Weathersbee, P. S.; Olsen, L. K.; and Lodge, J. R. 1977. "Caffeine and Pregnancy: A Retrospective Survey." *Postgraduate Medicine* 62(3):64–69.

25. Smith, B. E.; Gaub, M. L.; and Moya, F. 1965. "Investigations into the Teratogenic Effects of Anesthetic Agents: The Fluorinated Agents." *Anesthesiology* 26:260–61.

26. Butcher, R. E.; Vorhees, C. V.; and Kimmel, C. A. 1972. "Learning Impairment from Maternal Salicylate Treatment in Rats." *Nature; New Biology* 236:211–12.

27. Auletta, F. J. 1971. "Effect of Epinephrine on Implantation and Foetal Survival in the Rabbit." *Journal of Reproduction and Fertility* 27:281–85.

28. Morris, J. M. 1970. "Postcoital Antifertility Agents and Their Teratogenic Effect." *Contraception* 2:85–97.

29. Hodach, R. J.; Gilbert, E. F.; and Fallon, J. F. 1974. "Aortic Arch Anomalies Associated with Administration of Epinephrine in Chick Embryos." *Teratology* 9:203–9.

30. McColl, J. D.; Globus, M.; and Robinson, S. 1965. "Effect of Some Therapeutic Agents on the Developing Rat Fetus." *Toxicology and Applied Pharmacology* 7:409–17.

31. Tuchmann-Duplessis, H., and Mercier-Parot, L. 1954. "L'influence de la cortisone sur la gestation et le développement post natal du rat." *Comptes Rendus Hebdomadaires des Séances de l'Académie des Sciences. D: Sciences Naturelles* (Paris) 289:1689.

32. Johnstone, E. E., and Franklin, R. R. 1964. "Assay of Progestins for Fetal Virilizing Properties Using the Mouse. *Obstetrics and Gynecology* 23:359–62.

33. Loosli, R.; Loustalot, P.; Schalch, W. R.; Sievers, K.; and Stenger, E. G. 1964. "Joint Study in Teratogenicity Research, Preliminary Communication." *Proceedings of the European Society for Study of Drug Toxicity* 4:214–17.

34. Georges, A., and Denef, J. 1968. "Les anomalies digitales: Manifestations tératogéniques des dérivés xanthiques chez le rat." *Archives Internationales de Pharmacodynamie et de Therapie* 172: 219–22.

35. Scher, J.; Hailey, D. M.; and Beard, R. W. 1972. "The Effects of Diazepam on the Fetus." *Journal of Obstetrics and Gynaecology of the British Commonwealth* 79:635–38.

36. Dornhorst, A. C., and Young, I. M. 1952. "The Action of Adrenaline and Noradrenaline on the Placental and Foetal Circulations in the Rabbit and Guinea-pig." *Journal of Physiology* 118:282–88.

37. Vorhees, C. V.; Brunner, R. L.; and Butcher, R. E. 1979. "Psychotropic Drugs as Behavioral Teratogens." *Science* 205:1220–25.

38. Rothman, K. J.; Fyler, D. C.; Goldblatt, A.; and Kreidberg, M. B. 1979. "Exogenous Hormones and Other Drug Exposures of

Children with Congenital Heart Disease." *American Journal of Epidemiology* 109:433–39.

39. Morgan, I. 1978. "Metronidazole Treatment in Pregnancy." *International Journal of Gynaecology and Obstetrics* 15:501–2.

40. Woo, D., and Hoar, R. M. 1972. " 'Apparent Hydronephrosis' as a Normal Aspect of Renal Development in Late Gestation of Rats: The Effect of Methyl Salicylate." *Teratology* 6:191–96.

41. Kasirsky, G., and Lombardi, L. 1970. "Comparative Teratogenic Study of Various Corticoid Ophthalmics." *Toxicology and Applied Pharmacology* 16:773–78.

42. Naranjo, P., and Naranjo, E. 1968. "Embryotoxic Effects of Antihistamines." *Arzneimittel-Forschung* 18:188–95.

43. Corbett, T. H.; Beaudoin, A. R.; Cornell, R. G.; Endres, J. L.; and Page, A. 1974. "Effects of Low Concentrations of Methoxyflurane on Rat Pregnancy." *Teratology* 9:A15–A16.

44. Tuchman-Duplessis, H., and Mercier-Parot, L. 1958. "Influence d'un sulfamide hypoglycémiant, l'aminophénurobutane BZ55, sur la gestation de la ratte." *Comptes Rendus Hebdomadaires des Séances de l'Académie des Sciences. D: Sciences Naturelles* (Paris) 246:156.

45. Donarin, A. 1964. "Noradrenaline and the Foetal Heart." *Lancet* 1:756.

46. Hosoya, E.; Tokunaga, Y.; and Maruyama, D. 1967. "Studies on the Effects of Morphine Addiction upon the Fertility and Malformation in Rats and Mice." *Proceedings of the Congenital Anomalies Research Association of Japan* 7:63.

47. Takaya, M. 1965. "Teratogenic Effects of Antibiotics." *Osaka Shiritsu Daigaku Igaky Zasshi (Journal of the Osaka City Medical Center)* 14:107 (in Japanese).

48. Grollman, A., and Grollman, E. F. 1962. "The Teratogenic Induction of Hypertension." *Journal of Clinical Investigation* 41:710–14.

49. Wilson, J. G. 1971. "Use of Rhesus Monkeys in Teratological Studies." *Federation Proceedings* 30:104–9.

50. Wharton, R. S.; Wilson, A. I.; Mazze, R. I.; Baden, J. M.; and Rice, S. A. 1979. "Fetal Morphology in Mice Exposed to Halothane." *Anesthesiology* 51:532–37.

51. Buchan, P. C. 1979. "Pathogenesis of Neonatal Hyperbilirubinaemia after Induction of Labour with Oxytocin." *British Medical Journal* 2:1255–57.

52. Tanaka, S.; Kuwamura, T.; Kawashima, K.; Nakaura, S.; Nagao, S.; and Omori, Y. 1972. "Effects of Salicylic Acid and Ace-

Appendix C 147

tylsalicylic Acid on the Fetuses and Offspring of Rats." *Teratology* 6:121.

53. Bertrand, M.; Girod, J.; and Rigaud, M. F. 1970. "Ectrodactylie provoquée par la caféine chez les rongeurs. Rôle des facteurs spécifiques et génétiques." *Comptes Rendus des Séances de la Société de Biologie et des ses Filiales* (Paris) 164:1488.

54. Petrie, R. H.; Yeh, S-Y; Murata, U.; Paul, R. H.; Hon, E. H.; Barron, B. A.; and Johnson, R. J. 1978. "The Effect of Drugs on Fetal Heart Rate Variability." *American Journal of Obstetrics and Gynecology* 130:294–99.

55. Baxter, H., and Fraser, F. C. 1950. "Reduction of Congenital Defects in Offspring of Female Mice Treated with Cortisone." *McGill Medical Journal* 19:245.

56. Fink, B. R.; Shepard, T. H.; and Blandeau, R. J. 1967. "Teratogenic Activity of Nitrous Oxide." *Nature* 214:146–48.

57. Collins, T. F. X.; Hansen, W. H.; and Keeler, H. V. 1971. "Effect of Methyl salicylate on Rat Reproduction." *Toxicology and Applied Pharmacology* 18:755–65.

58. Olivecrona, H. 1964. "Embryo-Destroying Effect of Injected Phenobarbital in the Mouse." *Acta Anatomica* 58:217–21.

59. Smith, B. E.; Usubiaga, L. E.; and Lehrer, S. B. 1971. "Cleft Palate Induced by Halothane Anesthesia in C-57 Black Mice." *Teratology* 4:242.

60. Bedrick, A. D., and Ladda, R. L. 1978. "Epidermal Growth Factor Potentiates Cortisone-Induced Cleft Palate in the Mouse." *Teratology* 17:13–18.

61. Walker, B. E., and Patterson, A. 1974. "Induction of Cleft Palate in Mice by Tranquilizers and Barbiturates." *Teratology* 10:159–63.

62. Moore, D. O.; Bridenbaugh, L. D.; Thompson, G. E.; Balfour, R. I.; and Horton, W. G. 1978. "Bupivacaine: A Review of 11,080 Cases." *Anesthesie Analgesie Reanimation* 57:42–53.

63. Adamsons, K.; Mueller-Heuback, E.; and Myers, R. E. 1971. "Production of Fetal Asphyxia in the Rhesus Monkey by Administration of Catecholamines to the Mother." *American Journal of Obstetrics and Gynecology* 109:248–62.

64. Giroud, A.; Loustalot, P.; Madjerek, Z.; Millen, J. W.; Overbeck, G. A.; Somers, G. F.; Theiss, E.; Tuchmann-Duplessis, H.; and Woollam, D. H. M. 1966. "The Evaluation of Drugs for Foetal Toxicity and Teratogenicity in the Rat (Collaborative study by sixteen laboratories)." *Proceedings of the European Society for the Study of Drug Toxicity* 7:216.

65. Peterson. W. F.; Stauch, J. E.; and Ryder, C. D. 1966. "Metronidazole in Pregnancy." *American Journal of Obstetrics and Gynecology* 94:343–49.

66. Lewis, R. B., and Schulman, J. D. 1973. "Influence of Acetylsalicylic Acid, an Inhibitor of Prostaglandin Synthesis, on the Duration of Human Gestation and Labour." *Lancet* 2:1159–61.

67. Shoro, A. A. 1972. "Club-Foot and Intra-uterine Growth Retardation Produced by Tubocurarine Chloride in the Rat Fetus." *Journal of Anatomy* 111:506–8.

68. Earley, P. A., and Hayden, J. 1964. "Effect of Acetylsalicylic Acid on Foetal Rabbits." *Lancet* 1:763.

69. Palm, P. E.; Arnold, E. P.; Rachwall, P. C.; Leyczek, J. C.; Teague, K. W.; and Kensler, C. J. 1978. "Evaluation of the Teratogenic Potential of Fresh-Brewed Coffee and Caffeine in the Rat." *Toxicology and Applied Pharmacology* 44:1–16.

70. Larsson, K. S. 1962. "Studies on the Closure of the Secondary Palate. IV. Autoradiographic and Histochemical Studies of Mouse Embryos from Cortisone-Treated Mothers." *ACTA Morphologica Neerlando-Scandinavica* 4:369–86.

71. Jacobs, R. M. 1971. "Failure of Muscle Relaxants to Produce Cleft Palate in Mice." *Teratology* 4:25–30.

72. Zellers, J. E., and Gautieri, R. F. 1977. "Evaluation of Teratogenic Potential Codeine Sulfate in CF-1 Mice." *Journal of Pharmaceutical Sciences* 66:1727–31.

73. Tanimura, T.; Owaki, Y.; and Nishimura, H. 1967. "Effect of Administration of Thiopental Sodium to Pregnant Mice upon the Development of Their Offspring." *Okajimas Folia Anatomica Japonica* 43:219.

74. Geretto, P. 1973. "Acão teratogenica do fluotano no rato." *Revista brasileira de Anestesiologia* 23:17.

75. Davies, D. P.; Gomersall, R.; Robertson, R.; Gray, O. P.; and Turnbull, A. C. 1973. "Neonatal Jaundice and Maternal Oxytocin Infusion." *British Medical Journal* 3:476–77.

76. Ishikawa, S.; Gilbert, E. F.; Bruyere, Jr., H. J.; and Cheung, M. O. 1978. "Aortic Aneurysm Associated with Cardiac Defects in Theophylline Stimulated Chick Embryos." *Teratology* 18:23–30.

77. Eneroth, G.; Eneroth, P.; Forsberg, U.; Grant, C. A.; and Gustafsson, J. A. 1971. "Clomiphene-Induced Hydraminios and Fetal Cataracts in Rats Inhibited by Progesterone." *Teratology* 4:487. (Abstract)

78. Zimmerberg, B.; Charap, A. D.; and Glick, S. D. 1974. "Be-

havioral Effects of in Utero Administration of Morphine." *Nature* (London) 247:376–77.

79. Beard, R. W. 1962. "Response of Human Foetal Heart and Maternal Circulation to Adrenaline and Noradrenaline." *British Medical Journal* 1:443–46.

80. Eriksson, M. 1971. "Salicylate-induced Foetal Damage during Late Pregnancy in Mice: A Comparison between Sodium Salicylate, Acetylsalicylic Acid and Salicylsalicylic Acid." *Acta Pharmacologica et Toxicologica* 29:250–55.

81. Emerson, J. L.; Thompson, D. J.; Strebing, R. J.; Gerbig, C. G.; and Robinson, V. B. 1971. "Teratogenic Studies on 2,4,5-Trichlorophenoxyacetic Acid in the Rat and Rabbit." *Food and Cosmetics Toxicology* 9:395–404.

82. Love, E. J.; Kinch, R. A. H.; and Stevenson, J. A. F. 1964. "The Effect of Protamine Zinc Insulin on the Outcome of Pregnancy in the Normal Rat." *Diabetes* 13:44–48.

83. Braxy, J. E., and Pupkin, M. F. 1979. "Effects of Maternal Isoxsuprine Administration on Preterm Infants." *Journal of Pediatrics* 94:444–48.

84. Geber, W. F., and Schramm, L. C. 1975. "Congenital Malformations of the Central Nervous System Produced by Narcotic Analgesics in the Hamster." *American Journal of Obstetrics and Gynecology* 123:705–13.

85. Sethi, A., and Chaudhury, R. R. 1970. "Effect of Adrenergic Receptor-Blocking Drugs in Pregnancy in Rats." *Journal of Reproduction and Fertility* 21:551–54.

86. Iuliucci, J. D., and Gautieri, R. F. 1971. "Morphine-induced Fetal Malformations. II. Influence of Histamine and Diphenhydramine." *Journal of Pharmaceutical Sciences* 60:420–24.

87. Schardein, J. L.; Blatz, A. T.; Woosley, E. T.; and Kaump, D. H. 1969. "Reproduction Studies on Sodium Meclofenamate in Comparison to Aspirin and Phenylbutazone." *Toxicology and Applied Pharmacology* 15:46–55.

88. Friedler, G., and Cochin, J. 1972. "Growth Retardation in Offspring of Female Rats Treated with Morphine Prior to Conception." *Science* 175:654–55.

89. Fainstat, T. 1954. "Cortisone-induced Congenital Cleft Palate in Rabbits." *Endocrinology* 55:502–8.

90. Davis, M.E., and Plotz, E. J. 1954. "The Effects of Cortisone Acetate on Intact and Adrenalectomized Rats during Pregnancy." *Endocrinology* 54:384–95.

91. Smithberg, M., and Runner, M. N. 1963. "Teratogenic Effects of Hypoglycemic Treatments in Inbred Strains of Mice." *American Journal of Anatomy* 113:479–89.

92. Boucher, D., and Delost, P. 1964. "Développement post-natal des descendants issus de mères traitées par la pénicilline au cours de la gestation chez la souris." *Comptes Rendus des Séances de la Société de Biologie et des ses Filiales* (Paris) 158:528–32.

93. King. C. T. G.; Weaver, S. A.; and Narrod, S. A. 1965. "Antihistamines and Teratogenicity in the Rat." *Journal of Pharmacology and Experimental Therapeutics* 147:391–98.

94. McCormack, S., and Clark, J. H. 1979. "Clomid Administration to Pregnant Rats Causes Abnormalities of the Reproductive Tract in Offspring and Mothers." *Science* 204:629–31.

95. Reinisch, J. M.; Simon, N. G.; Karow, W. G.; and Gandelman, R. 1978. "Prenatal Exposure to Prednisone in Humans and Animals Retards Intrauterine Growth." *Science* 202:436–38.

96. Kameswaran, L.; Pennefather, J. N.; and West, G. B. 1962. "Possible Role of Histamine in Rat Pregnancy." *Journal of Physiology* 164:138–49.

97. Fujii, T., and Nishimura, H. 1969. "Teratogenic Actions of Some Methylated Xanthines in Mice." *Okajimas Folia Anatomica Japonica* 46:167.

98. Steele, W. J., and Johannesson, T. 1975. "Effects of Prenatally-administered Morphine on Brain Development and Resultant Tolerance to the Analgesic Effect of Morphine in Offspring of Morphine-treated rats." *Acta Pharmacologica Et Toxicologica* (Copenhagen) 36:243–56.

99. Beuker, E. D., and Platner, W. S. 1956. "Effect of Cholinergic Drugs on Development of Chick Embryo." *Proceedings of the Society for Experimental Biology and Medicine* 91:539–43.

100. Bertone, L. L., and Monie, I. W. 1965. "Teratogenic Effect of Methyl Salicylate and Hypoxia in Combination." *Anatomical Record* 151:443.

101. Bowman, R. E., and Smith, R. F. 1977. "Behavioral and Neurochemical Effects of Prenatal Halothane." *Environmental Health Perspective* 21:189–93.

102. Shapiro, S.; Heinonen, O. P.; Siskind, V.; Kaufman, D. W.; Monson, R. R.; and Slone, D. 1977. "Antenatal Exposure to Doxylamine Succinate and Dicyclomine Hydrochloride (Benedectin) in Relation to Congenital Malformations, Perinatal Mortality Rate, Birth Weight, and Intelligence Quotient Score." *American Journal of Obstetrics and Gynecology* 128:480–85.

103. Jeffares, M. J. 1977. "A Multifactorial Survey of Neonatal Jaundice." *British Journal of Obstetrics and Gynaecology* 84:452–55.

104. Johnson, W. E. 1971. "Fetal Loss from Anesthesia and Surgical Trauma in the Rabbit." *Toxicology and Applied Pharmacology* 18:773–79.

105. Temma, K.; Nishioeda, R.; Yoshida, Y.; Kaga, C.; and Kondo, H. 1978. "Effects of Repeated Morphine Treatment upon Maintenance of Pregnancy and Fetal Development in Rats." *Kitasato Archives of Experimental Medicine* 51:44–46.

106. Shabanah, E. H.; Tricomi, V.; and Suarez, J. R. 1969. "Fetal Environment and Its Influence on Fetal Development." *Surgery, Gynecology and Obstetrics* 129:556–64.

107. Baxi, L. V.; Petrie, R. H.; and James, L. S. 1979. "Human Fetal Oxygenation following Paracervical Block." *American Journal of Obstetrics and Gynecology* 135:1109–12.

108. Miller, F. C.; Quesnel, G.; Petrie, R. H.; Paul, R.H.; and Hon, E. H. 1978. "The Effects of Paracervical Block on Uterine Activity and Beat-to-Beat Variability of the Fetal Heart Rate." *American Journal of Obstetrics and Gynecology* 130:284–88.

109. Novitt, A. D., and Gilani, S. H. 1979. "Abnormal Embryogenesis Induced by Thiopental." *Journal of Clinical Pharmacology* 19:697–700.

110. Speert, H. 1940. "The Placental Transmission of Sulfanilamide and Its Effects upon the Fetus and Newborn." *Bulletin of the Johns Hopkins Hospital* 66:139–55.

111. Chomette, G. 1955. "Entwicklungsstörungen nach Insulinschock beim trächtigen Kaninchen." *Beitraege Zur Pathologischen Anatomie Und Zur Allgemeinen Pathologie* 115:439–51.

112. James, L. F.; Lazer, V. A.; and Binns, W. 1966. "Effects of Sublethal Doses of Certain Minerals on Pregnant Ewes and Fetal Development." *American Journal of Veterinary Research.* 27:132–35.

113. Aarskog, D. 1975. "Association between Maternal Intake of Diazepam and Oral Cleft." *Lancet* 2:921.

114. Vieira, E. 1979. "Effect of the Chronic Administration of Nitrous Oxide 0.5% to Gravid Rats." *British Journal of Anaesthesia* 51:283–87.

115. Gatling, R. R. 1962. "The Effect of Sympathomimetic Agents on the Chick Embryo." *American Journal of Pathology* 40:113–27.

116. Schardein, J. L.; Hentz, D. L.; Petrere, J. A.; and Kurtz, S. M. 1971. "Teratogenesis Studies with Diphenhydramine HCl." *Toxicology and Applied Pharmacology* 18:971.

117. Andrade, A. T. L.; Guimaraes, C. S.; and Guerra, M. O. 1972. "The 'In Vitro' Effects of Clomiphene Citrate on 6-day Rabbit Blastocysts and Their Subsequent 'In Vivo' Development." *Fertility and Sterility*. 23:841–46.

118. Rothberg, R. M.; Rieger, C. H. L.; Hill, J. H.; Danielson, J.; and Matadial, L. 1978. "Cord and Maternal Serum Meperidine Concentrations and Clinical Status of the Infant." *Biology of the Neonate* 33:80–89.

119. Auroux, M. 1973. "Influence de certaines substances médicamenteuses sur le développment tardif du système nerveux central du rat. Altération des capacités d'apprentissage de la progéniture par administration de phénobarbital à la mère." *Comptes Rendus des Séances de la Société de Biologie et des ses Filiales* (Paris) 167:797–801.

120. Brown, D. M.; Harper, K. H.; Palmer A. K.; and Tesh, S. A. 1968. "Effect of Antibiotics upon Pregnancy in the Rabbit." *Toxicology and Applied Pharmacology* 12:295.

121. Giurgea, M., and Puigdevall, J. 1968. "Maternal and Foetal Toxicity of Some Diphenylmethane Piperazine Derivatives." *Proceedings of the European Society for the Study of Drug Toxicity* 9:134–43.

122. Sullivan, F. M., and McElhatton, P. R. 1977. "A Comparison of the Teratogenic Activity of the Antiepileptic Drugs Carbamazepine, Clonazepam, Ethosuximide, Phenobarbital, Phenytoin, and Primidone in Mice." *Toxicology and Applied Pharmacology* 40:365–78.

123. Shelesnyak, M. C., and Davies, A. M. 1955. "Disturbance of Pregnancy in Mouse and Rat by Systemic Antihistaminic Treatment." *Proceedings of the Society for Experimental Biology and Medicine* 89:629–32.

124. Courtney, K. D., and Valerio, D. A. 1968. "Teratology in the Macaca Mulatta." *Teratology* 1:163–72.

125. Goldman, A. S., and Yakovac, W. C. 1965. "Teratogenic Action in Rats of Reserpine Alone and in Combination with Salicylate and immobilization." *Proceedings of the Society for Experimental Biology and Medicine* 118:857–62.

126. Wier, K. 1965. "Effect on the Weights of Fetuses and Fetal Lymphoid Organs of Adrenalin Given to Rabbits at a Critical Period of Pregnancy: Observations on Spontaneous and Induced Runting." *Anatomical Record* 153:373–76.

127. Mineshita, T.; Hasegawa, Y.; Yoshida, T.; Kozen, T.; Maeda, T.; Sakaguchi, I.; and Yamamoto, A. 1970. "Teratological

Effects of Dextropropoxyphene Napsylate on Foetuses and Suckling Young of Mice and Rats." *Oyo Yakuri* 4:1031–38.

128. Lapointe, R., and Harvey, E. B. 1964. "Salicylamide-induced Anomalies in Hamster Embryos." *Journal of Experimental Zoology* 156:197–99.

129. Landauer, W. 1947. "Insulin-induced Abnormalities of the Beak, Extremities and Eyes in Chickens." *Journal of Experimental Zoology* 105:145–72.

130. McColl, J. D.; Globus, M.; and Robinson, S. 1963. "Drug Induced Skeletal Malformations in the Rat." *Experientia* (Basel) 19:183–84.

131. Obbink, H. J. K., and Dalderup, L. M. 1964. "Effect of Acetylsalicylic Acid on Foetal Mice and Rats." *Lancet* 1:565.

132. Miyamoto, T., and Nagahama, M. 1967. "Experimental Studies of Congenital Hydrops Induced by Acetyl Salicylate (Aspirin) in Rats." *Proceedings of the Congenital Anomalies Research Association of Japan* 7:63.

133. Revesz, C.; Chappel, C. I.; and Gaudry, R. 1960. "Masculinization of Female Fetuses in the Rat by Progestational Compounds." *Endocrinology* 66:140–44.

134. Cliff, M. M., and Reynolds, S. R. M. 1959. "A Dose-Stress Response of Adrenaline Affecting Fetuses at a Critical Time in Pregnant Rabbits." *Anatomical Record* 134:379–84.

135. Palahniuk, R. J.; Doig, G. A.; Johnson, G. N.; and Pash, M. P. 1980. "Maternal Halothane Anesthesis Reduces Cerebral Blood Flow in the Acidotic Sheep Fetus." *Anesthesia and Analgesia* 59:35–39.

136. Persaud, T. V. N. 1965. "Tier experimentelle Untersuchungen zur Frage der teratogenen Wirkung von Barbituraten." *Acta Biologica et Medica Germanica* 14:89.

137. Angervall, L., and Martinsson, A. 1969. "Overweight in Offspring of Cortisone-treated Pregnant Rats." *Acta Endocrinologica* 60:36–46.

138. Shabanah, E. H.; Tricomi, V.; and Suarez, J. R. 1969. "Effect of Epinephrine on Fetal Growth and the Length of Gestation." *Surgery, Gynecology and Obstetrics* 129:341–43.

139. Collins, E., and Turner, G. 1973. "Salicylates and Pregnancy." *Lancet* 2:1494.

140. Jacobsen, L.; Kruse, V.; and Träff, B. 1970. "Eksperimentelle studier over halotans mulige teratogene effekt." *Nordisk Medicin* 84:941–44.

141. Szabo, K. T.; Free, S. M.; Birkhead, H. A.; Kang, Y. J.; Alston, E.; and Henry, M. 1971. "The Embryotoxic and Teratogenic Effects of Various Agents in the Fetal Mouse and Rabbit." *Toxicology and Applied Pharmacology* 19:371–72.

142. Chernoff, N., and Garbowski, C. T. 1971. "Responses of the Rat Foetus to Maternal Injections of Adrenaline and Vasopressin." *British Journal of Pharmacology* 43:270–78.

143. Scanlon, J. W.; Brown, W. U.; Weiss, J. B.; Alper, M. H. 1974. "Neurobehavioral Responses of Newborn Infants after Maternal Epidural Anesthesia." *Anesthesiology* 40:121–28.

144. Davis, W. M., and Lin, C. H. 1972. "Prenatal Morphine Effects on Survival and Behavior of Rat Offspring." *Research Communications in Chemical Pathology and Pharmacology* 3:205–14.

145. Harpel, H. S., Jr., and Gautieri, R. F. 1968. "Morphine-induced Fetal Malformations. I. Exencephaly and Axial Skeletal Fusions." *Journal of Pharmaceutical Sciences* 57:1590–97.

146. Smith, B. E.; Gaub, M. L.; and Moya, F. 1965. "Teratogenic Effects of Anesthetic Agents: Nitrous Oxide." *Anesthesia and Analgesia—Current Researches* 44:726–32.

147. Saxén, I., and Saxén, L. 1975. "Association between Maternal Intake of Diazepam and Oral Clefts." *Lancet* 2:498.

148. Brinsmade, A. B. 1957. "Entwicklungsstörungen am Kaninchenembryo nach Glukosemangel beim trächtigen Muttertier." *Beitraege Zur Pathologischen Anatomie Und Zur Allgemeinen Pathologie* 117:140–53.

149. Beall, J. R. 1972. "Study of the Teratogenic Potential of Diazepam and SCH 12041." *Canadian Medical Association Journal* 106:1061.

150. Brinsmade, A.; Büchner, F.; and Rübsaamen, H. 1956. "Missbildungen am Kaninchenembryo durch Insulininjektion beim Muttertier." *Naturwissenschaften* 43:259.

151. Ornoy, A., and Horowitz, A. 1972. "Postnatal Effects of Maternal Hypercortisonism on Skeletal Development in Newborn Rats." *Teratology* 6:153–58.

152. Fujii, T.; Sasaki, H.; and Nishimura, H. 1969. "Teratogenicity of Caffeine in Mice Related to Its Mode of Administration." *Japanese Journal of Pharmacology* 19:134–38.

153. Kennedy, L. A., and Persaud, T. V. 1978. "Pentobarbital Intoxication in the Pregnant Rat." *Research Communications in Chemical Pathology and Pharmacology* 20:179–82.

154. Picon, L. 1967. "Effect of Insulin on Growth and Biochemical Composition of the Rat Fetus." *Endocrinology* 81:1419–21.

155. Safra, M. J., and Oakley, G. P. 1975. "An Association of

Cleft Lip with or without Cleft Palate and Prenatal Exposure to Valium." *Lancet* 2:478–79.

156. Lopez-Escobar, G., and Fridhandler, L. 1969. "Studies of Clomiphene Effects on Rabbit Embryo Development and Biosynthetic Activity." *Fertility and Sterility* 20:697–714.

157. Corby, D. G., Zirbel, C. L.; Gibson, M. S.; and Schulman, I. 1973. "Effect of Antenatal Drug Administration on Aggregation of Platelets of Newborn Infants." *Clinical Toxicology* 6:300–301.

158. Bertrand, M; Schwam, E.; Frandon, A.; Vagne, A.; and Alary, J. 1965. "Sur un effet tératogène systématique et spécifique de la caféine chez les rongeurs." *Comptes Rendus des Séances de la Société de Biologie et des ses Filiales* 159:2199, 2202.

159. Basford, A. B., and Fink, B. R. 1968. "The Teratogenicity of Halothane in the Rat." *Anesthesiology* 29:1167–73.

160. Nelson, M. M., and Forfar, J. O. 1971. "Associations between Drugs Administered during Pregnancy and Congenital Abnormalities of the Fetus." *British Medical Journal* 1:523–27.

161. Stoklosa, E.; Kosmider, S.; Brezegowy, A.; and Mikolajczyk, G. 1971. "Experimental Studies on the Influence of Penicillin and Streptomycin Administered during Pregnancy on the Fetal Rat Liver." *Patologia Polska* 22:653 (in Polish).

162. Jost, A. 1953. "Degenerescence des extremites du foetus de rat provoquée par l'adrenaline." *Comptes Rendus Hebdomadaires Des Séances de L'Academie des Sciences. D: Sciences Naturelles* 236:1510–12.

163. Trasler, D. G. 1965. "Aspirin-induced Cleft Lip and Other Malformations in Mice." *Lancet* 1:606.

164. Sivasuriya, M.; Tan, K. L.; Salmon, Y. M.; and Karim, S. M. 1978. "Neonatal Serum Bilirubin Levels in Spontaneous and Induced Labour." *British Journal of Obstetrics and Gynaecology* 85:619–23.

165. Miller, R. P., and Becker, B. A. 1975. "Teratogenicity of Oral Diazepam and Diphenylhydantoin in Mice." *Toxicology and Applied Pharmacology* 32:53–61.

166. Friedman, E. A.; Sachtleben, M. R.; and Wallace, A. K. 1979. "Infant Outcome following Labor Induction." *American Journal of Obstetrics and Gynecology* 133:718–22.

167. Butcher, R. E. 1978. "Halothane—A Behavioral Teratogen?" *Anesthesiology* 49:308–9.

168. Crist, T., and Hulka, J. F. 1970. "Influence of Maternal Epinephrine on Behavior of Offspring." *American Journal of Obstetrics and Gynecology* 106:687–91.

169. Vieira, E.; Cleaton-Jones, P.; Austin, J. C.; Moyes, D. G.;

and Shaw, R. 1980. "Effects of Low Concentrations of Nitrous Oxide on Rat Fetuses." *Anesthesie, Analgesie, Reanimation* 59:175–77.

170. Lane, G. A.; Nahrwold, M. L.; Tait, A. R.; Taylor-Busch, M.; Cohen, P. J.; and Beaudoin, A. R. 1980. "Anesthetics as Teratogens: Nitrous Oxide is Fetotoxic, Xenon Is Not." *Science* 210:899–901.

171. Stenchever, M. A., and Parks, K. J. 1975. "Some Effects of Diazepam on Pregnancy in the Balb/C Mouse." *American Journal of Obstetrics and Gynecology.* 121:765–69.

172. King, C. T. G., and Howell, J. 1966. "Teratogenic Effect of Buclizine and Hydroxyzine in the Rat and Chlorcyclizine in the Mouse." *American Journal of Obstetrics and Gynecology* 95:109–11.

173. Erisson, M., and Larsson, K. S. 1968. "Premature Birth Induced in Mice by Salicylate." *Nature* (London) 220:385.

174. Miller, R. P., and Becker, B. A. 1973. "The Teratogenicity of Diazepam Metabolites in Swiss-Webster Mice." *Toxicology and Applied Pharmacology* 25:453. (Abstract)

175. Zimmerman, E. F., and Bowen, D. 1972. "Distribution and Metabolism of Triamcinolone Acetonide in Mice Sensitive to Its Teratogenic Effects." *Teratology* 5:57–69.

176. D'Souza, S. W.; Black, P.; MacFarlane, T.; and Richards, B. 1979. "The Effect of Oxytocin in Induced Labour on Neonatal Jaundice." *British Journal of Obstetrics and Gynaecology* 86:133–38.

177. Smithells, R. W., and Sheppard, S. 1978. "Teratogenicity Testing in Humans: A Method Demonstrating Safety of Bendectin." *Teratology* 17:31–35.

178. Saxén, I. 1974. "Cleft Palate and Maternal Diphenhydramine Intake." *Lancet* 1:407–8.

179. Wood, B.; Culley, P.; Roginski, C.; Powell, J.; and Waterhouse, J. 1979. "Factors Affecting Neonatal Jaundice." *Archives of Disease in Childhood* 54:111–15.

180. Corby, D. G., and Schulman, I. 1971. "The Effects of Antenatal Drug Administration on Aggregation of Platelets of Newborn Infants." *Journal of Pediatrics* 79:307–13.

181. Tuchmann-Duplessis, H.; Mottot, G.; Hiss, D.; and Rosner, I. 1974. "Prolongation de la durée de gestation et de parturition chez le rat traité par l'aspirine." *Therapie* 29:877–82.

182. Flowers, C. E.; Rudolph, A. J.; and Desmond, M. M. 1969. "Diazepam as an Adjunct in Obstetric Analgesia." *Obstetrics and Gynecology* 34:68–81.

183. Baba, T.; Nagahama, M.; Akiyama, N.; and Miki, T. 1966. "Experimental Production of Malformations Due to Acetyl Salicylate and Phenyl Salicylate in Rats." *Osaka City Medical Journal* 12:23.

184. Scanlon, J. W.; Ostheimer, G. W.; Lurie, A. O.; Brown, W. U., Jr.; Weiss, J. B.; and Alper, M. H. 1976. "Neurobehavioral Responses and Drug Concentrations in Newborns after Maternal Epidural Anesthesia with Bupivacaine." *Anesthesiology* 45:400–405.

185. Chang, L. W.; Dudley, A. W., Jr.; Katz, J.; and Martin, A. H. 1974. "Nervous System Development following In Utero Exposure to Trace Amounts of Halothane." *Teratology* 9:A15.

186. Setälä, K., and Nyyssönen, O. 1964. "Hypnotic Sodium Pentobarbital as a Teratogen for Mice." *Naturwissenschaften* 51:413.

187. Jost, A.; Roffi, J.; and Cowitat, M. 1969. "Congenital Amputations Determined by the BR Gene and Those Induced by Adrenalin Injection in the Rabbit Fetus." In *Limb Development and Deformity: Problems of Evaluation and Rehabilitation,* edited by C. A. Swinyard, 187–99. Springfield, Ill.: C. C. Thomas.

188. Johannesson, T., and Becker, B. A. 1972. "The effects of Maternally Administered Morphine on Rat Foetal Development and Resultant Tolerance to the Analgesic Effect of Morphine." *Acta Pharmacologica et Toxicologica* 31:305–13.

189. Walker, B. E., and Patterson, A. 1978. "Palate Development after Fetal Tongue Removal in Cortisone-treated Mice." *Teratology* 17:51–55.

190. Fahim, M. S.; Hall, D. G.; Jones, T. M.; Fahim, Z.; and Whitt, F. D. 1970. "Drug-steroid Interaction in the Pregnant Rat, Fetus and Neonate." *American Journal of Obstetrics and Gynecology* 107:1250–58.

191. Friedman, L; Lewis, P. J.; Clifton, P.; and Bulpitt, C. J. 1978. "Factors Influencing the Incidence of Neonatal Jaundice." *British Medical Journal* 1:1235–37.

192. Bleyer, W. A., and Breckenridge, R. T. 1970. "Studies on the Detection of Adverse Drug Reactions in the Newborn. II. The Effects of Prenatal Aspirin on Newborn Hemostasis." *Journal of the American Medical Association* 213:2049–53.

193. Suzuki, M. R. 1970. "Effects of Oral Cyclofenil and Clomiphene, Ovulation Inducing Agents on Pregnancy and Fetuses in Rats." *Oyo Yakuri* 4:645–51.

194. Mellin, G. W. 1975. "Report on Prochlorperazine Utilization during Pregnancy from the Fetal Life Study Data Bank." *Teratology* 11:28A (Abstract).

195. Roux, C. 1959. "Action tératogène de la prochlorpérazine." *Archives Francaises de Pédiatrie* 16:968–71.

196. Bollert, J. A.; Gray, J. E.; Highstrete, J. D.; Moran, J.; Purmalis, B. P.; and Weaver, R. N. 1974. "Teratogenicity and Neo-

natal Toxicity of Clindamycin 2-Phosphate in Laboratory Animals."
Toxicology and Applied Pharmacology 27:322–29.

197. Suchowsky, G. K., and Junkmann, K. 1961. "A Study of the
Virilizing Effect of Progestogens on the Female Rat Fetus." *Endocrinology* 68:341–49.

198. Bovet-Nitti, F.; Bignami, G.; and Bovet, D. 1963. "Antihistamine Drugs on Rat Pregnancy: Effects of Pyrilamine and Meclizine." *Life Sciences* 5:303–10.

199. Ferrill, H. W. 1943. "Effect of Chronic Insulin Injections on
Reproduction in White Rats." *Endocrinology* 32:449–50.

200. Becker, R. F.; Flannagan, E.; and King, J. E. 1958. "The
Fate of Offspring from Mothers Receiving Sodium Pentobarbital before Delivery." *Neurology* 8:776–82.

201. Ream, J. R., Jr.; Weingarten, P. L.; and Pappas, A. M.
1970. "Evaluation of the Prenatal Effects of Massive Doses of Insulin
in Rats." *Teratology* 3:29–32.

202. Ridgway, L. P., and Karnofsky, D. A. 1952. "The Effects of
Metals on the Chick Embryo: Toxicity and Production of Abnormalities in Development." *Annals of the New York Academy of Sciences*
55:203–15.

203. Föllmer, W., and Kramer. 1951. "Zur Toxikologie der Sulfonamide. Der Einfluss von Sulfonamiden auf die Schwangerschaft."
Archiv für Gynaekologie 179:123–35.

204. Merkow, A. J.; McGuinness, G. A.; Erenberg, A.; and Kennedy, R. L. 1980. "The Neonatal Neurobehavioral Effects of Bupivacaine, Mepivacaine, and 2-Chloroprocaine Used for Pudendal Block."
Anesthesiology 52:309–12.

205. Lichtenstein, H.; Guest, G. M.; and Warkany, J. 1951. "Abnormalities in Offspring of White Rats Given Protamin Zinc Insulin
During Pregnancy." *Proceedings of the Society for Experimental Biology and Medicine* 78:398–402.

206. Walker, B. E. 1965. "Cleft Palate Produced in Mice by
Human-Equivalent Dosage with Triamcinolone." *Science* 149:862–63.

207. Nishimura, H., and Nakai, K. 1960. "Congenital Malformations in Offspring of Mice Treated with Caffeine." *Proceedings of the
Society for Experimental Biology and Medicine* 104:140–42.

208. Tanimura, T. 1972. "Effects on Macaque Embryos of
Drugs Reported or Suspected to Be Teratogenic to Humans." *Acta
Endocrinological Supplementum* (Copenhagen) Suppl. No. 166,
293–308.

209. Moriguchi, M.; Fujita, M.; Sato, H.; Hata, T.; Yamashita,
Y.; and Koeda, Y. 1976. "Effects of Viccillin Injection on Fetuses."
Personal Communication. Cited in H. Nishimura and T. Tanimura

(1976), *Clinical Aspects of the Teratogenicity of Drugs,* p. 123, Excerpta Medica, Amsterdam.

210. Tronick, E.; Wise, S.; Als, H.; Adamson, L.; Scanlon, J.; and Brazelton, T. B. 1976. "Regional Obstetric Anesthesia and Newborn Behavior: Effect over the First Ten Days of Life." *Pediatrics* 58:94–100.

211. Kato, T., and Kitagawa, S. 1973. "Production of Congenital Anomalies in Fetuses of Pregnant Rats and Mice Treated with Various Sulfonamides." *Senten Ijo* 13:7.

212. Schifferli, P., and Caldeyro-Barcia, R. 1973. "Effects of Atropine and Beta-Adrenergic Drugs on Heart Rate of the Human Fetus." In *Fetal Pharmacology,* edited by L. O. Boreus, 259–79. New York: Raven Press.

213. Zawoiski, E. J. 1976. "Prevention of Caffeine-induced Cleft Palate by L-Glutamic Acid." *Toxicology and Applied Pharmacology* 35(1):123–28.

214. Keeler, R. F., and Binns, W. 1968. "Teratogenic Compounds of *Veratrum Californicum* (Durand). V. Comparison of Cyclopian Effects of Steroidal Alkaloids from the Plant and Structurally Related Compounds from Other Sources." *Teratology* 1:5–10.

215. Zawoiski, E. J. 1980. "Effect of L-Glutamic Acid on Glucocorticoid-induced Cleft Palate in Gestating Albino Mice. *Toxicology and Applied Pharmacology* 56(1):23–27.

216. Singhi, S., and Singh, M. 1979. "Pathogenesis of Oxytocin-induced Neonatal Hyperbilirubinaemia." *Archives of Disease in Childhood* 54(5):400–402.

217. Teramo, K.; Benowitz, N.; Heymann, M. A.; and Rudolph, A. M. 1976. "Gestational Differences in Lidocaine Toxicity in the Fetal Lamb." *Anesthesiology* 44(2):133–38.

218. Bornschein, R. L.; Hastings, L.; and Manson, J. M. 1980. "Behavioral Toxicity in the Offspring of Rats Exposed to Dichlormethane (DCM) prior to and/or during Gestation." *Toxicology and Applied Pharmacology* 52:29–37.

219. Wharton, R. S.; Sievenpiper, T. S.; and Mazze, R. I. 1980. "Developmental Toxicity of Methoxyflurane in Mice." *Anesthesie, Analgesie, Reanimation* 59(6):421–25.

220. Pope, W.; Halsey, M.; Lansdown, A.; Simmonds, A.; and Bateman, P. 1978. "Fetotoxicity in Rats following Chronic Exposure to Halothane, Nitrous Oxide, or Methoxyflurane." *Anesthesiology* 48:11–16.

221. Beall, J. R., and Klein, M. F. 1977. "Enhancement of Aspirin-induced Teratogenicity by Food Restriction in Rats." *Toxicology and Applied Pharmacology* 39(3):489–95.

222. Schoenfeld, N.; Epstein, O.; Nemesh, L.; Rosen, M.; and Atsmon, A. 1978. "Effects of Propranolol during Pregnancy and Development of Rats. I. Adverse Effects during Pregnancy." *Pediatric Research* 12(7):747–50.

223. Conway, D. I.; Read, M. D.; Bauer, C.; and Martin, R. H. 1976. "Neonatal Jaundice—A Comparison between Intravenous Oxytocin and Oral Prostaglandin E2." *Journal of International Medical Research* 4(4):241–46.

224. Pruyn, S. C.; Phelan, J. P.; and Buchanan, G. C. 1979. "Long-term Propranolol Therapy in Pregnancy: Maternal and Fetal Outcome." *American Journal of Obstetrics and Gynecology* 135(4): 485–89.

225. O'Shea, K. S., and Kaufman, M. H. 1980. "Neural Tube Closure Defects following In Vitro Exposure of Mouse Embryos to Xylocaine." *Journal of Experimental Zoology* 214(2):235–38.

226. Wiener, P. C.; Hogg, M. I. J.; and Rosen, M. 1977. "Effects of Naloxone on Pethidine-induced Neonatal Depression." *British Medical Journal* 2:228–31.

227. Gould, S. R.; Mountrose, U.; Brown, D. J.; Whitehouse, W. L.; and Barnardo, D. E. 1974. "Influence of Previous Oral Contraception and Maternal Oxytocin Infusion on Neonatal Jaundice." *British Medical Journal* 3:228.

228. Shah, R. M., and Kilistoff, A. 1976. "Cleft Palate Induction in Hamster Fetuses by Glucocorticoid Hormones and Their Synthetic Analogues." *Journal of Embryology and Experimental Morphology* 36(1):101–8.

229. Fujii, T. 1976. "Mitigation of Caffeine-induced Fetopathy in Mice by Pretreatment with Beta-Adrenergic Blocking Agents." *Japanese Journal of Pharmacology* 26(6):751–56.

230. Woo, D. C., and Hoar, R. M. 1972. "Apparent Hydronephrosis as a Normal Aspect of Renal Development in Late Gestation of Rats: The Effects of Methyl Salicylate." *Teratology* 6:191–96.

231. Boylan, P. 1976. "Oxytocin and Neonatal Jaundice." *British Medical Journal* 2(6035):564–65.

232. Gilani, S. H., and Silvestri, A. 1977. "The Effect of Propranolol upon Chick Embryo Cardiogenesis." *Experimental Cell Biology* 45(3–4):158–66.

233. Ballas, S.; Toaff, M. E.; and Toaff, R. 1976. "Effects of Intravenous Meperidine and Meperidine with Promethazine on Uterine Activity and Fetal Heart Rate during Labor." *Israel Journal of Medical Sciences* 12(10):1141–47.

234. Shah, R. M.; Burdett, D. N.; and Donaldson, D. 1979. "The

Effects of Nitrous Oxide on the Developing Hamster Embryo." *Canadian Journal of Physiology and Pharmacology* 57(11):1229–32.

235. Silbermann, M., and Levitan, S. 1979. "Corticosteroid-induced Mandibular Growth Retardation and Palatal Malformation in the ICR Mouse Fetus." *Journal of Anatomy* 128(4):747–65.

236. Robertson, R. T.; Allen, H. L.; and Bokelman, D. L. 1979. "Aspirin: Teratogenic Evaluation in the Dog." *Teratology* 20(2):313–20.

237. Wright, R. G.; Shnider, S. M.; Levinson, G.; Rolvin, S. H.; and Parer, J. T. 1981. "The Effect of Maternal Administration of Ephedrine on Fetal Heart Rate and Variability." *Obstetrics and Gynecology* 57(6):734–38.

238. Crowell, D. H.; Sharma, S. D.; Philip, A. G.; Kapuniai, L. E.; Waxman, S. H.; and Hale, R. W. 1980. "Effects of Induction of Labor on the Neurophysiologic Functioning of Newborn Infants." *American Journal of Obstetrics and Gynecology* 136(1):48–53.

239. Shapiro, S.; Siskind, V.; Monson, R. R.; Heinonen, O. P.; Kaufman, D. W., and Slone, D. 1976. "Perinatal Mortality and Birth-Weight in Relation to Aspirin Taken during Pregnancy." *Lancet* 1:1375–76.

240. Granat, M.; Borochowitz, Z.; Berger, A.; and Sharf, M. 1981. "Bilirubin and Protein Concentration in Cord Blood after Spontaneous Versus Induced Labor. Correlation to Neonatal Hyperbilirubinemia." *Journal of Perinatal Medicine*. 9(1):27–34.

241. Rosenkranz, P. G.; Gordon, D. R.; Speck, W. T.; and Rosenkranz, H. S. 1980. "Developmental Abnormalities in the American Sea Urchin Induced by Povidone-Iodine, a Widely Used Vaginal Antiseptic." *Mutation Research* 77(4):387–90.

242. Foote, W. D.; Foote, W. C.; and Foote, L. H. 1968. "Influence of Certain Natural and Synthetic Steroids in Genital Development in Guinea Pigs." *Fertility and Sterility* 19:606–15.

243. Brazy, J. E.; Little, V.; and Grimm, J. 1981. "Isoxsuprine in the Perinatal Period. II. Relationships between Neonatal Symptoms, Drug Exposure, and Drug Concentration at the Time of Birth." *Journal of Pediatrics* 98(1):146–51.

244. Popova, S.; Virgieva, T.; Atanasova, J.; Atanasov, A.; and Sahatchiev, B. 1979. "Embryotoxicity and Fertility Study with Halothane Subanaesthetic Concentration in Rats." *Acta Anaesthesiologica Scandinavica* 23(6):505–12.

245. Stephen, G. W.; Cooper, L. V.; and Harvey, D. 1976. "The Effect of Narcotic and Narcotic-Antagonist Drugs in the Newborn Rabbit." *British Journal of Anaesthesia* 48(7): 635–38.

246. Gerhardt, T.; Bancalari, E.; Cohen, H,; and Macias-Loza, M. 1977. "Respiratory Depression at Birth—Value of Apgar Score and Ventilatory Measurements in Its Detection." *Journal of Pediatrics* 90(6):971–75.

247. Chew, W. C., and Swann, I. L. 1977. "Influence of Simultaneous Low Amniotomy and Oxytocin Infusion and Other Maternal Factors on Neonatal Jaundice: A Prospective Study." *British Medical Journal* 1:72–73.

248. Barlow, S. M.; Knight, A. F.; and Sullivan, F. M. 1980. "Diazepam-induced Cleft Palate in the Mouse: The Role of Endogenous Maternal Corticosterone." *Terotology* 21(2):149–55.

249. Piotrowski, J. 1969. "Experimental Studies on the Effect of Some Steroid Hormones on the Development of the Rabbit Fetus. II." *Przeglad Lekarski* 25:322–24.

250. Fritz, H.; Muller, D.; and Hess, R. 1976. "Comparative Study of the Teratogenicity of Phenobarbitone, Diphenylhydantoin and Carbamazepine in Mice." *Toxicolology* 14(3):281–85.

251. Elovaara, E.; Hemminki, K.; and Vainio, H. 1979. "Effects of Methylene Chloride, Trichloroethane, Trichloroethylene, Tetrachloroethylene and Toluene on the Development of Chick Embryos." *Toxicology* 12(2):111–19.

252. Cordero, J. F.; Oakley, G. P.; Greenberg, F.; and James, L. M. 1981. "Is Bendectin a Teratogen?" *Journal of the American Medical Association* 245(22):2307–10.

253. Nelson, M. M., and Forfar, J. O. 1971. "Associations between Drugs Administered during Pregnancy and Congenital Abnormalities of the Fetus." *British Medical Journal* 1:523–27.

254. Cockroft, D. L., and Coppola, P. T. 1977. "Teratogenic Effects of Excess Glucose on Head-Fold Rat Embryos in Culture." *Teratology* 16(2):141–46.

255. Chew, W. C. 1977. "Neonatal Hyperbilirubinaemia: A Comparison between Prostaglandin E2 and Oxytocin Inductions." *British Medical Journal* 2:679–80.

256. Lubawy, W. C., and Burris Garrett, R. J. 1977. "Effects of Aspirin and Acetaminophen on Fetal and Placental Growth." *Journal of Pharmaceutical Sciences* 66:111–13.

257. Halsey, M. J.; Green, C. J.; Monk, S. J.; et al. 1981. "Maternal and Paternal Chronic Exposure to Enflurane and Halothane: Foetal and Histological Changes in the Rat." *British Journal of Anaesthesia* 53(3):203–15.

258. Brackbill, Y.; Kane, J.; Manniello, R. L.; and Abramson, D. 1974. "Obstetrical Meperidine Usage and Assessment of Neonatal Status." *Anesthesiology* 40:116–20.

259. Lerner, L. J.; DePhillipo, M.; Yiacas, E.; Brennan, D.; and Borman, A. 1962. "Comparison of the Acetophenone Derivative of 16a, 17-a-Dihydroxyprogesterone with Other Progestational Steroids for Masculinization of the Rat Fetus." *Endocrinology* 71:448–51.

260. Sawyer, R.; Hendrickx, A.; Osburn, B.; Terrell, T.; and Anderson, J. 1977. "Abnormal Morphology of the Fetal Monkey (Macaca Mulatta) Thymus Exposed to a Corticosteroid." *Journal of Medical Primatology* 6(3):145–150.

261. Beazley, J. M., and Alderman, B. 1975. "Neonatal Hyper-bilirubinaemia following the Use of Oxytocin in Labor." *British Journal of Obstetrics and Gynaecology* 82:265.

262. Khera, K. S. 1976. "Teratogenicity Studies with Methotrexate, Aminopterin, and Acetylsalicylic Acid in Domestic Cats." *Teratology* 14(1):21–27.

263. Hardin, B. D., and Manson, J. M. 1980. "Absence of Dichloromethane Teratogenicity with Inhalation Exposure in Rats." *Toxicology and Applied Pharmacology* 52(1):22–28.

264. Slone, D.; Siskind, V.; Heinonen, O. P.; Monson, R. R.; Kaufman, D. W.; and Shapiro, S. 1976. "Aspirin and Congenital Malformations." *Lancet* 1:1373–75.

265. Singhi, S. , and Singh, M. 1979. "Transplacental Asymptomatic Hyponatremia following Oxytocin Infusion during Labour." *Indian Journal of Medical Sciences* 70:55–57.

266. Adams, C. E.; Hay, M. F.; and Lutwak-Mann, C. 1961. "The Action of Various Agents upon the Rabbit Embryo." *Journal of Embryology and Experimental Morphology* 9:468–91.

267. Scanlon, J. W.; Suzuki, K.; Shea, E.; and Tronick, E. 1978. "Clinical and Neurobehavioral Effects of Repeated Intrauterine Exposure to Oxytocin: A Prospective Study." *American Journal of Obstetrics and Gynecology* 132(3):294–96.

268. Berry, C. L., and Nickols, C. D. 1979. "The Effects of Aspirin on the Development of the Mouse Third Molar. A Potential Screening System for Weak Teratogens." *Archives of Toxicology* 42(3):185–90.

269. Kennedy, G. L., Jr.; Smith, S. H.; Keplinger, M. L.; and Calandra, J. C. 1976. "Reproductive and Teratologic Studies with Halothane." *Toxicology and Applied Pharmacology* 35(3):467–74.

270. Belfrage, P.; Boréus, L. O.; Hartvig, P.; Irestedt, L.; and Raabe, N. 1981. "Neonatal Depression after Obstetrical Analgesia with Pethidine. The Role of the Infection-Delivery Time Interval and of the Plasma Concentrations of Pethidine and Norpethidine." *Acta Obstetrica et Gynecologica Scandinavica* 60(1):43–49.

271. "Teratogenicity of nitrous oxide." 1981. *FDA Drug Bulletin* 11(1):7.

272. Hendrickx, A. G.; Sawyer, R. H.; Terrell, T. G.; Osburn, B. I.; Henrickson, R. V.; and Steffek, A. J. 1975. "Teratogenic Effects of Triamcinolone on the Skeletal and Lymphoid Systems in Nonhuman Primates." *Federation Proceedings* 34:1661–65.

273. Brice, J. E.; Moreland, T. A.; and Walker, C. H. 1979. "Effects of Pethidine and Its Antagonists on the Newborn." *Archives of Disease in Childhood.* 54(5):356–61.

274. Freysz, H.; Willard, D.; Lehr, A.; Messer, J.; and Boog, G. 1977. "A Long Term Evaluation of Infants Who Received a Beta-Mimetic Drug while In Utero." *Journal of Perinatal Medicine* 5(2):94–99.

275. O'Connor, M.C.; Murphy, H.; and Dalrymple, I. J. 1979. "Double Blind Trial of Ritodrine and Placebo in Twin Pregnancy." *British Journal of Obstetrics and Gynaecology* 2:947–49.

276. Gray, J. H.; Cudmore, D. W.; Luther, E. R.; Martin, T. R.; and Gardner, A. J. 1978. "Sinusoidal Fetal Heart Rate Pattern Associated with Alphaprodine Administration." *Obstetrics and Gynecology* 52(6):678–81.

277. Belsky, D. H. 1982. "Statistical Observations on the Elective Induction of Labor with Oxytocin." *Journal of the American Osteopathic Association* 81(8):524–30.

278. Kenepp, N. B.; Kumar, S.; Shelley, W. C.; Stanley, C. A.; Gabbe, S. G.; and Gutsche, B. B. 1982. "Foetal and Neonatal Hazards of Maternal Hydration with 5% Dextrose before Caesaren Section." *Lancet* 1:1150–52.

279. Rasch, D. K.; Huber, P. A.; Richardson, C. J.; L'Hommedieu, C. S.; Nelson, T. E.; and Reddi, R. 1982. "Neurobehavioral Effects of Neonatal Hypermagnesemia." *Journal of Pediatrics* 100(2):272–76.

280. Guerriero, F. J., and Fox, K. A. 1976. "Benzodiazepines and Reproduction of Swiss-Webster Mice." *Research Communications in Chemical Pathology and Pharmacology* 13(4):601–10.

281. Nemeth, I.; Szeleczki, T.; and Boda, D. 1981. "Hyperbilirubinemia and Urinary D-Glucaric Acid Excretion in Premature Infants following Antepartum Dexamethasone Treatment." *Journal of Perinatal Medicine* 9(1):35–39.

282. Shah, R. M., and Kilistoff, A. 1976. "Cleft Palate Induction in Hamster Fetuses by Glucocorticoid Hormones and their Synthetic Analogues." *Journal of Embryology and Experimental Morphology* 36(1):101–8.

283. Rosenberg, L.; Mitchell, A. A.; Shapiro, S.; and Slone, D. 1982. "Selected Birth Defects in Relation to Caffeine-containing

Beverages." *Journal of the American Medical Association* 247(10):1429–32.

284. Stuart, M. J.; Gross, S. J.; Elrad, H.; and Graeber, J. E. 1982. "Effects of Acetylsalicylic-Acid Ingestion on Maternal and Neonatal Hemostasis." *New England Journal of Medicine* 307 (15):909–12.

285. Morelock, S.; Hingson, R.; Kayne, H.; Dooling, E.; Zuckerman, B.; Day, N.; Alpert, J. J.; and Flowerdew, G. 1982. "Bendectin and Fetal Development. A Study of Boston City Hospital." *American Journal of Obstetrics and Gynecology* 142(2):209–13.

286. Buttar, H. S. 1980. "Effects of Chlordiazepoxide on the Pre- and Postnatal Development of Rats. *Toxicology* 17(3):311–21.

287. Wong, Y. C.; Beardsmore, C. S.; and Silverman, M. 1982. "Antenatal Dexamethasone and Subsequent Lung Growth." *Archives of Disease in Childhood* 57(7):536–38.

288. Sanfacon, R.; Possmayer, F.; and Harding, P. G. 1977. "Dexamethasone Treatment of the Guinea Pig Fetus: Its Effects on the Incorporation of 3H-Thymidine into Deoxyribonucleic Acid." *American Journal of Obstetrics and Gynecology* 127(7):745–52.

289. Lee, F.; Nelson, N.; Faiman, C.; Choi, N. W.; and Reyes, F. I. 1982. "Low-Dose Corticoid Therapy for Anovulation: Effect upon Fetal Weight." *Obstetrics and Gynecology* 60(3):314–17.

290. Rumack, C. M.; Guggenheim, M. A.; Rumack, B. H.; Peterson, R. G.; Johnson, M. L.; and Braithwaite, W. R. 1981. "Neonatal Intracranial Hemorrhage and Maternal Use of Aspirin." *Obstetrics and Gynecology* 58(5 Suppl):52S–56S.

291. Stefani, S. J.; Hughes, S. C.; Shnider, S. M.; Levinson, G.; Abboud, T. K.; Henriksen, E. H.; Williams, V.; and Johnson, J. 1982. "Neonatal Neurobehavioral Effects of Inhalation Analgesia for Vaginal Delivery." *Anesthesiology* 56(5):351–55.

References

Abboud, T. K.; Khoo, S. S.; Miller, F.; Doan, T.; and Henriksen, E. H. 1982. "Maternal, Fetal and Neonatal Responses after Epidural Anesthesia with Bupivacaine, 2-Chloroprocaine, or Lidocaine." *Anesthesia and Analgesia* 61:638–43.

Aleksandrowicz, M. K., and Aleksandrowicz, D. R. 1974. "Obstetrical Pain Relieving Drugs as Predictors of Infant Behavior Variability." *Child Development* 45:935–45.

Alfidi, R. J. 1971. "Informed Consent: A Study of Patient Reaction." *Journal of the American Medical Association* 216:1325–29.

American Society of Hospital Pharmacists. 1976. Statement on Pharmacist-Conducted Patient Counseling. *American Journal of Hospital Pharmacy* 33:644.

Appelbaum, P. S., and Roth, L. H. 1982. "Treatment Refusal in Medical Hospitals." In *Making Health Care Decisions,* Report of the President's Commission for the Study of Ethical Problems in Medicine and Biomedical and Behavioral Research, App. D, 411–76. Washington, D.C.: U.S. Government Printing Office.

Armitage, K. J.; Schneiderman, L. J.; and Bass, R. A. 1979. "Response of Physicans to Medical Complaints in Men and Women." *Journal of the American Medical Association* 241:2186–87.

Banta, D., and Thacker, S. 1979. "Electronic Fetal Monitoring. Is It of Benefit?" *Birth and the Family Journal* 6:237–49.

Baraka, A.; Maktabi, M; and Noueihid, R. 1982. "Epidural Meperidine-Bupivacaine for Obstetric Analgesia." *Anesthesia and Analgesia* 61:652–56.

Baraka, A.; Noueihid, R; and Hajj, S. 1981. "Intrathecal Injection of Morphine for Obstetric Analgesia." *Anesthesiology* 54:136–40.

Belsey, E. M.; Rosenblatt, D. B.; Lieberman, B. A.; Redshaw, M.; Caldwell, J.; Notarianni, L.; Smith, R. L.; and Beard, R. W. 1981. "The Influence of Maternal Analgesia on Neonatal Behaviour: I. Pethidine." *British Journal of Obstetrics and Gynaecology* 88:398–406.

Bertakis, K. D. 1977. "The Communication of Information from

Physician to Patient: A Method for Increasing Patient Retention and Satisfaction." *Journal of Family Practice* 5:217–22.

Bonta, B. W.; Gagliardi, J. O.; Williams, V.; and Warshaw, J. B. 1979. "Naloxone Reversal of Mild Neurobehavioral Depression in Normal Newborn Infants after Routine Obstetric Analgesia." *Journal of Pediatrics* 94:102–5.

Boreham, P., and Gibson, D. 1978. "The Informative Process in Private Medical Consultations: A Preliminary Investigation." *Social Science and Medicine* 12:409–16.

Borgstedt, A. D., and Rosen, M. G. 1968. "Medication during Labor Correlated with Behavior and EEG of the Newborn." *American Journal of Diseases of Children* 115:21–24.

Boyd, J. R.; Covington, T. R.; Stanaszek, W. F.; and Coussons, R. T. 1974. "Drug Defaulting. Part II: Analysis of Noncompliance Patterns." *American Journal of Hospital Pharmacy* 31:485–91.

Brackbill, Y. 1976. "Long Term Effects of Obstetrical Anesthesia on Infant Autonomic Function." *Developmental Psychobiology* 9(4):353–58.

Brackbill, Y. 1979. "Obstetrical Medication and Infant Behavior." In *Handbook of Infant Development*, edited by J. D. Osofsky, 76–125. New York: John Wiley and Sons.

Brackbill, Y.; Kane, J.; Manniello, R. L.; and Abramson, D. 1974a. "Obstetrical Meperidine Usage and Assessment of Neonatal Status." *Anesthesiology* 40:116–20.

Brackbill, Y.; Kane, J.; Manniello, R. L.; and Abramson, D. 1974b. "Obstetrical Premedication Usage and Outcome." *American Journal of Obstetrics and Gynecology* 118:377–84.

Brackbill, Y.; Rice, J.; and Young, D. 1984. *Birth Trap*. St. Louis, Mo.: C. V. Mosby.

Brazelton, T. B. 1961. "Psychophysiologic Reaction in the Neonate. II. The Effects of Maternal Medication on the Neonate and His Behavior." *Journal of Pediatrics* 58:513–18.

Brazelton, T. B. 1973. "Neonatal Behavioral Assessment Scale." *Clinics in Developmental Medicine*, No. 50. London: Heineman.

Brazelton, T. B.; Tryphonopoulou, Y.; and Lester, B. M. 1979. "A Comparative Study of the Behavior of Greek Neonates." *Pediatrics* 63:279–85.

Brower, K. R.; Crowell, D. H.; Leung, P.; and Cashman, T. M. 1978. "Neonatal Electroencephalographic Patterns as Affected by Maternal Drugs Administered during Labor and Delivery." *Anesthesia and Analgesia* 57:303–6.

Brown, J. V.; Bakeman, R.; Snyder, P. A.; Fredrickson, W. T.;

Morgan, S. T.; and Hepler, R. 1975. "Interactions of Black Inner-City Mothers with Their Newborn Infants." *Child Development* 46:677–86.

Brown, N. A., and Fabro, S. 1983. "The Value of Animal Teratogenicity Testing for Predicting Human Risk." *Clinical Obstetrics and Gynecology* 26:467–77.

Brown, W. A.; Manning, T.; and Grodin, J. 1972. "The Relationship of Antenatal and Perinatal Psychologic Variables to the Use of Drugs in Labor." *Psychosomatic Medicine* 34:119–27.

Busacca, M.; Gementi, P.; Gambini, E.; Lenti, C.; Meschi, F.; and Vignali, M. 1982. "Neonatal Effects of the Administration of Meperidine and Promethazine to the Mother in Labor. Double Blind Study." *Journal of Perinatal Medicine* 10:48–51.

Clark, R. B.; Beard, A. G.; Greifenstein, F. E.; and Barclay, D. L. 1976. "Naloxone in the Parturient and Her Infant." *Southern Medical Journal* 69(5):570–78.

Colcher, I. S., and Bass, J. W. 1972. "Penicillin Treatment of Streptococcal Pharyngitis: A Comparison of Schedules and the Role of Specific Counseling." *Journal of the American Medical Association* 222:657–59.

Comstock, L. M.; Hooper, E. M.; Goodwin, J. M.; and Goodwin J. S. 1982. "Physician Behaviors That Correlate with Patient Satisfaction." *Journal of Medical Education* 57:105–12.

Conway, E., and Brackbill, Y. 1970. "Delivery Medication and Infant Outcome: An Empirical Study." In W. A. Bowes, Jr., Y. Brackbill, E. Conway, and A. Steinschneider. *Monographs of the Society for Research in Child Development, 35* (Serial No. 137), 24–34.

Corke, B. C. 1977. "Neurobehavioral Responses of the Newborn." *Anesthesia* 32:539–43.

Cruickshank, W. M. 1980. Foreword to *Learning Disabilities and Brain Function,* by W. H. Gades, v–vii. New York: Springer-Verlag.

Danziger, S. K. 1978. "The Uses of Expertise in Doctor-Patient Encounters during Pregnancy." *Social Science and Medicine* 12:359–67.

Datta, S.; Corke, B. C.; Alper, M. H.; Brown, W. U.; Ostheimer, G. W.; and Weiss, J. B. 1980. "Epidural Anesthesia for Cesarean Section: A Comparison of Bupivacaine, Chloroprocaine, and Etidocaine." *Anesthesiology* 51:48–51.

Doering, P. L., and Stewart, R. B. 1978. "The Extent and Character of Drug Consumption during Pregnancy." *Journal of the American Medical Association* 239:843–46.

Dubignon, J.; Campbell, D.; Curtis, M.; and Partington, M. 1969. "The Relation between Laboratory Measures of Sucking, Food Intake, and Perinatal Factors during the Newborn Period." *Child Development* 40:1107–20.

Eagly, A. H. 1983. "Gender and Social Influence: A Social Psychological Analysis." *American Psychologist* 38:971–81.

Egbert, L. D.; Battit, G. E.; Welch, C. E.; and Bartlett, M. K. 1964. "Reduction of Post Operative Pain by Encouragement and Instruction of Patients." *New England Journal of Medicine* 270:825–27.

Ehrenreich, B., and Ehrenreich, J. 1974. "Health Care and Social Control." *Social Policy,* May/June, 26–40.

Ehrenreich, B., and English, D. 1973. *Complaints and Disorders: The Sexual Politics of Sickness.* New York: Feminist Press.

Emde, R. N.; Swedberg, J.; and Suzuki, B. 1975. "Human Wakefulness and Biological Rhythms after Birth." *Archives of General Psychiatry* 32:780–83.

Erickson, J. D. 1981. "Epidemiology and Developmental Toxicology." In *Developmental Toxicology,* edited by C. A. Kimmel and J. Buelke-Sam, 289–301. New York: Raven Press.

Federman, E. J., and Yang, R. K. 1976. "A Critique of Obstetrical Pain-Relieving Drugs as Predictors of Infant Behavior Variability." *Child Development* 47:294–96.

Finger, S., and Simons, D. 1976. "Effects of Serial Lesions of Somatosensory Cortex and Further Neodecortication on Retention of a Rough-Smooth Discrimination in Rats." *Experimental Brain Research* 25:183–97.

Fitzpatrick, R. M., and Hopkins, A. 1981. "Patient's Satisfaction with Communication in Neurological Outpatient Clinics." *Journal of Psychosomatic Research* 25:329–34.

Fleckenstein, L.; Joubert, P.; Lawrence, R.; Patsner, B.; Mazzullo, J. M.; and Lasagna, L. 1976. "Oral Contraceptive Patient Information: A Questionnaire Study of Attitudes, Knowledge, and Preferred Information Sources." *Journal of the American Medical Association* 235:1331–36.

Frankfort, E. 1972. *Vaginal Politics.* New York: Quadrangle.

Friedman, C. M.; Greenspan, R.; and Mittleman, F. 1974. "The Decision-making Process and the Outcome of Therapeutic Abortion." *American Journal of Psychiatry* 131:1332–37.

Friedman, S. L.; Brackbill, Y.; Caron, A. J.; and Caron, R. F. 1978. "Obstetric Medication and Visual Processing in 4- and 5-Month-Old Infants." *Merrill-Palmer Quarterly* 24:111–28.

Gaddes, W. H. 1980. *Learning Disabilities and Brain Function.* New York: Springer-Verlag.

Garber, J., and Seligman, M. E. P. 1980. *Human Helplessness: Theory and Applications.* New York: Academic Press.

Gillette, J. L.; Byrne, T. J.; and Cranton, J. W. 1982. "Variables Affecting Patient Satisfaction with Health Care Services in the College Health Setting." *Journal of the American College Health Association* 30:167–70.

Gotsch, A. R., and Liguori, S. 1982. "Knowledge, Attitude, and Compliance Dimensions of Antibiotic Therapy with PPIs." *Medical Care* 20(6):581–93.

Gray, B. H. 1975. *Human Subjects in Medical Experimentation.* New York: Wiley.

Hallahan, D. P., and Cruickshank, W. M. 1973. *Psychoeducational Foundations of Learning Disabilities.* Englewood Cliffs, N. J.: Prentice-Hall.

Harris, L.; Boyle, J. M.; and Brounstein, P. J. 1982. "Views of Informed Consent and Decision Making: Parallel Surveys of Physicians and the Public." In *Making Health Care Decisions,* Report of the President's Commission for the Study of Ethical Problems in Medicine and Biomedical and Behavioral Research, App. B, 17–26. Washington D. C.: U. S. Government Printing Office.

Herman, E.; Miller-Klein, V.; and Ventre, F. 1979. "A Survey of Current Trends in Home Birth." In *Compulsory Hospitalization.* Marble Hill, Mo.: Napsac Reproductions.

Hill, R. M. 1973. "Drugs Ingested by Pregnant Women." *Clinical Pharmacology and Therapeutics* 14:654–59.

Hodgkinson, R.; Bhatt, M.; Grewal, G.; and Marx, G. F. 1978. "Neonatal Neurobehavior in the First 48 Hours of Life: Effect of the Administration of Meperidine with and without Naloxone in the Mother." *Pediatrics* 62:294–98.

Hodgkinson, R.; Bhatt, M.; Kim, S. S.; Grewal, G.; and Marx, G. F. 1978. "Neonatal Neurobehavioral Tests following Cesarean Section with General and Spinal Anesthesia." *American Journal of Obstetrics and Gynecology* 132:670–73.

Hodgkinson, R.; Bhatt, M.; and Wang, C. N. 1978. "Double-Blind Comparison of the Neurobehavior of Neonates following the Adminisration of Different Doses of Meperidine to the Mother." *Canadian Anaesthetists' Society Journal* 25:405–11.

Hodgkinson, R.; Marx, G. F.; Kim, S. S.; and Miclat, N. M. 1977. "Neonatal Neurobehavioral Tests following Vaginal Delivery under Ketamine, Thiopental and Extradural Anesthesia." *Anesthesia and Analgesia* 56:548–53.

Hodgkinson, R.; Wang, C. N.; and Marx, G. F. 1976. "Evaluation of the Effects of General Anaesthesia and Pethidine on Neurobehavioural Tests during the First 2 Days of Life." *Anaesthesia* 31:143–44.

Hollmen, A. I.; Jouppila, R.; Koivisto, M.; Maatta, L.; Pihlajaniemi, R.; Puukka, M.; and Rantakyla, P. 1978. "Neurologic Activity of Infants following Anesthesia for Cesarean Section." *Anesthesiology* 48:350–56.

Horowitz, F. D.; Ashton, J.; Culp, R.; Gaddis, E.; Levin, S.; and Reichmann, B. 1977. "The Effects of Obstetrical Medication on the Behavior of Israeli Newborn Infants and Some Comparisons with Uruguayan and American Infants." *Child Development* 48:1607–23.

Hughes, J. G.; Ehemann, B.; and Brown, V. A. 1948. "Electroencephalography of the Newborn: III. Brain Potentials of Babies Born of Mothers Given 'Seconal Sodium.' " *American Journal of Diseases of Children* 76:626–33.

Hughes, J. G.; Hill, F. S.; Green, C. R.; and Davis, B. C. 1950. "Electroencephalography of the Newborn: V. Brain Potentials of Babies Born of Mothers Given Meperidine Hydrochloride (Demerol Hydrochloride), Vinbarbital Sodium (Delvinal Sodium) or Morphine." *American Journal of Diseases of Children* 79:996–1007.

International Childbirth Education Association. 1981. Position Statement on Electronic Fetal Monitoring. *International Childbirth Education Association News* 20:4–6.

Iseroff, A. 1980. "Facilitation of Delayed Spontaneous Alternation Behavior in Adult Rats following Early Hydroxyzine Treatment: Differential Sensitivity in Late Infancy." *Psychopharmacology* 69:179–81.

Ivy, A. C. 1948. "The History and Ethics of the Use of Human Subjects in Medical Experiments." *Science* 108:1–5.

Janis, I. L. 1958. *Psychological Stress: Psychoanalytic and Behavioral Studies of Surgical Patients*. New York: Wiley.

Janis, I. L., and Mann, L. 1977. *Decision Making*. New York: Free Press.

Joyce, C. R. B.; Caple, G.; Mason, M.; Reynolds, E.; and Mathews, J. A. 1969. "Quantitative Study of Doctor-Patient Communication." *Quarterly Journal of Medicine* 38:183–94.

Kaufmann, C. L. 1982. "Medical Education and Physician-Patient Communication." In *Making Health Care Decisions*, Report of the President's Commission for the Study of Ethical Problems in

Medicine and Biomedical and Behavioral Research, App. I, 117–42. Washington, D. C.: U. S. Government Printing Office.

Kennedy, Donald. 1980. "Science and Health Regulation." *Journal of Dental Education* 44:473–77.

Kirke, P. N. 1980. "Mothers' Views of Obstetric Care." *British Journal of Obstetrics and Gynaecology* 87:1029–33.

Korsch, B. M., and Negrete, V. F. 1972. "Doctor-Patient Communication." *Scientific American* 222:66–74.

Kraemer, H.; Korner, A.; and Thoman, E. 1972. "Methodological Considerations in Evaluating the Influence of Drugs Used during Labor and Delivery on the Behavior of the Newborn." *Developmental Psychology* 6:128–34.

Kron, R. E.; Stein, M.; and Goddard, K. E. 1966. "Newborn Sucking Behavior Affected by Obstetric Sedation." *Pediatrics* 37:1012–16.

Langer, E., and Rodin, J. 1976. "The Effects of Choice and Enhanced Personal Responsibility for the Aged: A Field Experiment in an Institutional Setting." *Journal of Personality and Social Psychology* 34:191–98.

Lefcourt, H. M. 1976. *Locus of Control: Current Trends in Theory and Research.* New Jersey: Halsted Press.

Lefcourt, H. M., and Wine, J. 1969. "Internal Versus External Control of Reinforcement and the Development of Attention in Experimental Situations." *Canadian Journal of Behavioral Science* 1:167–81.

Lester, B. M.; Als, H.; and Brazelton, T. B. 1982. "Regional Obstetric Anesthesia and Newborn Behavior: A Reanalysis Toward Synergistic Effects." *Child Development* 53:687–92.

Ley, P.; Bradshaw, P. W.; Eaves, D. E.; and Walker, C. M. 1973. "A Method for Increasing Patients' Recall of Information Presented to Them." *Psychological Medicine* 3:217–20.

Ley, P.; Bradshaw, P. W.; Kincey, J. A.; and Atherton, S. T. 1976. "Increasing Patients' Satisfaction with Communications." *British Journal of Social and Clinical Psychology* 15:403–13.

Ley, P., and Spelman, M. S. 1967. *Communicating with the Patient.* London: Staples Press.

Ley, P.; Whitworth, M. A.; Skilbeck, C. E.; Woodward, R.; Pinsont, R. J. F. H.; Pike, L. A.; Clarkson, M. E.; and Clark, P. B. 1976. "Improving Doctor-Patient Communication in General Practice." *Journal of the Royal College of General Practitioners* 26:720–24.

Lidz, C. W., and Meisel, A. 1982. "Informed Consent and the Structure of Medical Care." In *Making Health Care Decisions,* Report of the President's Commission for the Study of Ethical Problems in

Medicine and Biomedical and Behavioral Research, App. C, 317–406. Washington, D. C.: U.S. Government Printing Office.

Lidz, C. W., and Roth, L. H. 1983. "The Signed Form—Informed Consent?" In *Solutions to Legal and Ethical Problems in Applied Social Research,* edited by R. F. Boruch et al. New York: Academic Press.

Lieberman, B. A.; Rosenblatt, D. B.; Belsey, E.; Packer, M.; Redshaw, M.; Mills, M.; Caldwell, J.; Notarianni, L.; Smith, R. L.; Williams, M.; and Beard, R. W. 1979. "The Effects of Maternally Administered Pethidine or Epidural Bupivacaine on the Fetus and Newborn." *British Journal of Obstetrics and Gynaecology* 86:598–606.

Lukes, S. 1974. *Power: A Radical View.* London: Macmillan.

Lund, P. C.; Cwik, J. C.; Gannon, R. T.; and Vassallo, H. G. 1977. "Etidocaine for Caesarean Section—Effects on Mother and Baby." *British Journal of Anaesthesia* 49:457–60.

MacDonald, E. T.; MacDonald, J. B.; and Phoenix, M. 1977. "Improving Drug Compliance after Hospital Discharge." *British Medical Journal* 2:618–21.

McCann, M. B., and Stare, F. J. 1967. "The Contribution of Animal Studies to Nutritional Discoveries That Have Benefited Both Animals and Man." *American Journal of Public Health* 57:1597–1604.

McGuinness, G. A.; Merkow, A. J.; Kennedy, R. L.; and Erenberg, E. A. 1978. "Epidural Anesthesia with Bupivacaine for Cesarean Section: Neonatal Blood Levels and Neurobehavioral Responses." *Anesthesiology* 49:270–73.

McKenney, J. M.; Slinling, J. M.; Henderson, H. R.; Devins, D.; and Barr, M. 1973. "The Effect of Clinical Pharmacy Services on Patients with Essential Hypertension." *Circulation* 48:1104–11.

McManus, K. A.; Brackbill, Y.; Woodward, L.; Doering, P.; and Robinson, D. 1982. "Consumer Information about Prenatal and Obstetric Drugs." *Women and Health* 7:15–29.

Mazis, M.; Morris, L. A.; and Gordon, E. 1978. "Patient Attitudes about Two Forms of Printed Oral Contraceptive Information." *Medical Care* 16:1045–54.

Meis, P. J.; Reisner, L. S.; Payne, T. F.; and Hobel, C. J. 1978. "Bupivacaine Paracervical Block: Effects on the Fetus and Neonate." *Obstetrics and Gynecology* 52:545–48.

Mendelsohn, R. 1979. *Confessions of a Medical Heretic.* Chicago: Contemporary Books.

Merkow, A. J.; McGuinness, G. A.; Erenberg, A.; and Kennedy, R. L. 1980. "The Neonatal Neurobehavioral Effects of Bupivacaine, Mepivacaine and 2-Chloroprocaine Used for Pudendal Block." *Anesthesiology* 52:309–12.

Michael, M., and Bordley, C. 1982. "Do Patients Want Access to Their Medical Records?" *Medical Care* 20:432–35.

Milgram, S. 1965. "Some Conditions of Obedience and Disobedience to Authority." *Human Relations* 18:57–76.

Milgram, S. 1974. *Obedience to Authority: An Experimental View.* New York: Harper and Row.

Mills, R. T., and Krantz, D. S. 1979. "Information, Choice, and Reactions to Stress: A Field Experiment in a Blood Bank with Laboratory Analogue." *Journal of Personality and Social Psychology* 37:608–20.

Mitscherlich, A., and Mielke, F. 1949. *Doctors of Infancy: The Story of the Nazi Medical Crimes.* Translated by H. Norden. New York: H. Schuman.

Moreau, T., and Birch, H. G. 1974. "Relationship between Obstetrical General Anesthesia and Rate of Neonatal Habituation to Repeated Stimulation." *Developmental Medicine and Child Neurology* 16:612–19.

Morris, L. A., and Kanouse, D. E. 1981. "Consumer Reactions to the Tone of Written Drug Information." *American Journal of Hospital Pharmacy* 38:667–71.

Morris, L. A., and Kanouse, D. E. 1982. "Informing Patients about Side Effects." *Journal of Behavioral Medicine* 5:363–73.

Morris, L. A.; Mazis, M.; and Gordon, E. 1977. "A Survey of the Effects of Oral Contraceptive Patient Information." *Journal of the American Medical Association* 238:2504–8.

Murray, A. D.; Dolby, R. M.; Nation, R. L.; and Thomas, D. B. 1981. "Effects of Epidural Anesthesia on Newborns and Their Mothers." *Child Development* 52:71–82.

Myers, E. D., and Calvert, E. J. 1973. "The Effect of Forewarning on the Occurrence of Side Effects and the Discontinuance of Medication in Patients on Amitriptyline." *British Journal of Psychiatry* 122:461–64.

Myers, E. D., and Calvert, E. J. 1976. "The Effects of Forewarning on the Occurrence of Side Effects and Discontinuance of Medication in Patients on Dothiepin." *Journal of International Medical Research* 4:237–40.

Nesheim, B. I.; Lindbaek, E.; Storm-Mathisen, I.; and Jenssen, H. 1979. "Neurobehavioral Responses of Infants after Paracervical Block during Labor." *Acta Obstetrica et Gynecologica Scandinavica* 58:41–44.

Norell, S. E. 1979. "Improving Medication Compliance: A Random-ised Clinical Trial." *British Medical Journal* 2:1031–33.

Ounsted, M. K.; Boyd, P. A.; Hendrick, A. M.; Mutch, L. M. M.; Simons, C. D.; and Good, F. J. 1978. "Induction of Labor by Different Methods in Primiparous Women II. Neurobehavioral Status of the Infants." *Early Human Development* 121:241–53.

Palahniuk, R. J.; Scatcliff, J.; Biehl, D.; Wiebe, H.; and Sankaran, K. 1977. "Maternal and Neonatal Effects of Methoxyflurane, Ni-trous Oxide and Lumbar Epidural Anesthesia for Cesarean Sec-tion." *Canadian Anesthetists' Society Journal* 24:586–96.

Parke, R. D.; O'Leary, S. E.; and West, S. 1972. "Mother-Father-Newborn Interaction: Effects of Maternal Medication, Labor, and Sex of Infant." *Proceedings of the 80th Annual Convention of the American Psychological Association,* 85–86.

Paulson, P. T.; Bauch, R.; Paulson, M. L.; and Zilz, D. A. 1976. "Medication Data Sheets—An Aid to Patient Education." *Drug Intelligence and Clinical Pharmacy* 10:448–53.

Pernick, M. S. 1982. "The Patient's Role in Medical Decisionmaking: A Social History of Informed Consent in Medical Therapy." In *Making Health Care Decisions,* Report of the President's Commis-sion for the Study of Ethical Problems in Medicine and Biomedical and Behavioral Research, App. E, 1–35. Washington, D.C.: U.S. Government Printing Office.

Phares, E. J. 1968. "Differential Utilization of Information as a Func-tion of Internal-External Control." *Journal of Personality* 36:649–62.

Pohl, J. M., and Fuller, S. S. 1980. "Perceived Choice, Social Inter-action and Dimensions of Morale of Residents in a Home for the Aged." *Research in Nursing and Health* 3:147–57.

President's Commission for the Study of Ethical Problems in Medi-cine and Biomedical and Behavioral Research. 1982. *Making Health Care Decisions. A Report on the Ethical and Legal Implica-tions of Informed Consent in the Patient-Practitioner Relationship.* Vol. 1. Washington D. C.: U.S. Government Printing Office.

Price, J. L. W. 1977. "The Patient's Morale." *Lancet* 1:533.

Prociuk, T. J., and Breen, L. J. 1977. "Internal-External Locus of Control and Information-Seeking in a College Academic Situa-tion." *Journal of Sociology and Psychology* 101:309–10.

PsyINFO Retrospective. 1982. *Learning and Communication Dis-orders. An Abstracted Bibliography, 1971–1980.* Washington D. C.: American Psychological Association.

Putt, A. M. 1970. "One Experiment in Nursing Adults with Peptic Ulcers." *Nursing Research* 19:484–94.

Richards, M. P. M., and Bernal, J. F. 1972. "An Observational Study of Mother-Infant Interaction." In *Ethological Studies of Child Behavior,* edited by N. B. Jones, 175–97. Cambridge, England: Cambridge University Press.

Robinson, H. J. 1967. "Animal Experimentation Leading to the Development of Drugs Benefiting Human Beings and Animals." *American Journal of Public Health* 57:1613–20.

Rodin, J.; Bohm, L. C.; and Wack, J. T. 1982. "Control, Coping, and Aging: Models for Research and Intervention." In *Applied Social Psychology Annual,* edited by L. Bickman, 3:153–80. Beverly Hills, Calif.: Sage.

Rodin, J., and Langer, E. 1977. "Long-Term Effect of a Control Relevant Intervention." *Journal of Personality and Social Psychology* 35:897–902.

Rooth, G.: Lysikiewicz, A.; Huch, R.; and Huch, A. 1983. "Some Effects of Maternal Pethidine Administration on the Newborn." *British Journal of Obstetrics and Gynaecology* 90:28–33.

Rosenberg, S. G. 1971. "Patient Education Leads to Better Care for Heart Patients." *Health Services and Mental Health Administration Health Reports* 86:793.

Rosenblatt, D. B.; Belsey, E. M.; Lieberman, B. A.; Redshaw, M.; Caldwell, J.; Notarianni, L.; Smith, R. L.; and Beard, R. W. 1981. "The Influence of Maternal Analgesia on Neonatal Behaviour: II. Epidural Bupivacaine." *British Journal of Obstetrics and Gynaecology* 88:407–13.

Ross, D. M., and Ross, S. A. 1982. *Hyperactivity: Current Issues, Research, and Theory.* 2d ed. New York: Wiley.

Rotter, J. B. 1966. "Generalized Expectancies for Internal Versus External Control of Reinforcement." *Psychological Monographs* 80:1–28.

Russo, E. J. 1977. "The Value of Unit Price Information." *Journal of Marketing Research* 14:193–201.

Russo, E. J.; Krieser, G.; and Miyashita, S. 1975. "An Effective Display of Unit Price Information." *Journal of Marketing* 39:11–19.

Ruzek, S. 1978. *The Women's Health Movement.* New York: Praeger Publishers.

Ryan, J., and McMahon, F. G. 1977. "Potential Effects on the Health Care System—2." *Drug Information Journal* (Supplement):75–79.

Saunderson, G. R. 1977. "The Effectiveness of Two Types of Pre-
paratory Messages on the Responses of Patients Undergoing Sig-
moidoscopy Examination." *Abstracts of Hospital Management
Studies* 14:246.

Scanlon, J. W.; Brown, W. U., Jr.; Weiss, J. B.; and Alper, M. H.
1974. "Neurobehavioral Responses of Newborn Infants after Maternal Epidural Anesthesia." *Anesthesiology* 40:121–28.

Scanlon, J. W.; Ostheimer, G. W.; Lurie, A. O.; Brown, W. U., Jr.;
Weiss, J. B.; and Alper, M. H. 1976. "Neurobehavioral Responses and Drug Concentrations in Newborns after Maternal Epidural Anesthesia with Bupivacaine." *Anesthesiology* 45:400–405.

Schultz, A. L.; Pardee, G. P.; and Ensinck, J. W. 1975. "Are Research Subjects Really Informed?" *Western Journal of Medicine*
123:76–80.

Schulz, R. 1976. "Effects of Control and Predictability on the Physical and Psychological Well-Being of the Institutionalized Aged."
Journal of Personality and Social Psychology 33:563–73.

Seeman, M. 1963. "Alienation and Learning in a Reformatory."
American Journal of Sociology 69:270–84.

Seeman, M., and Evans, J. W. 1962. "Alienation and Learning in a
Hospital Setting." *American Sociological Review* 27:772–83.

Seligman, M. E. P. 1975. *Helplessness: On Depression, Development,
and Death.* San Francisco: Freeman.

Seligman, M. E. P., and Miller, S. M. 1979. "The Psychology of
Power: Concluding Comments." In *Choice and Perceived Control,*
edited by L. C. Perlmutter and R. A. Monty. Hillsdale, N.H.: L.
Erlbaum Associates.

Seltzer, A.; Roncari, I.; and Garfinkel, P. 1980. "Effect of Patient
Education on Medication Compliance." *Canadian Journal of Psychiatry* 25:638–45.

Sharpe, T. R., and Mikeal, R. L. 1974. "Patient Compliance with
Antibiotic Regimens." *American Journal of Hospital Pharmacy*
31:479–84.

Shapiro, M. C.; Najman, J. M.; Chang, A.; Keeping, J. D.; Morri-
son, J.; and Western, J. S. 1983. "Information Control and the
Exercise of Power in the Obstetrical Encounter." *Social Science
and Medicine* 17:139–46.

Shaw, N. S. 1974. *Forced Labor: Maternity Care in the United States.*
New York: Pergamon Press.

Shnider, S. M.; Abboud T. K.; Levinson, G.; Wright, R. G.; Kim, S.;
Henriksen, E.; Hughes, S.; Roizen, M. F.; and Johnson, J. 1979.
"General Anesthesia for Cesarean Section: Maternal and Fetal

Norepinephrine Levels and Neonatal Neurobehavioral Status." *Anesthesiology* 53:5301.

Simons, D.; Puretz, J.; and Finger, S. 1975. "Effects of Serial Lesions of Somatosensory Cortex and Further Neodecortication on Tactile Retention in Rats." *Experimental Brain Research* 23:353–66.

Smoking and Health. Report of the Advisory Committee to the Surgeon General of the Public Health Service. 1964. Washington, D. C.: U.S. Department of Health, Education and Welfare, 182–89.

Standley, K.; Soule, A. B., III; Copans, S. A.; and Duchowny, M. S. 1974. "Local-Regional Anesthesia during Childbirth: Effect on Newborn Behaviors." *Science* 186:634–35.

Starr, P. 1982. *The Social Transformation of American Medicine.* New York: Basic Books.

Stechler, G. 1964. "Newborn Attention as Affected by Medication during Labor." *Science* 144:315–17.

Stefani, S. J.; Hughes, S. C.; Shnider, S. M.; Levinson, G.; Abboud, T. K.; Henriksen, E. H.; Williams, V.; and Johnson, J. 1982. "Neonatal Neurobehavioral Effects of Inhalation Analgesia for Vaginal Delivery." *Anesthesiology* 56:351–55.

Sudman, S., and Bradburn, N. M. 1974. *Response Effects in Surveys: A Review and Synthesis.* Chicago: Aldine.

Svarsted, B. L. 1976. "Physician-Patient Communication and Patient Conformity with Medical Advice." In *The Growth of Bureaucratic Medicine,* edited by D. Mechanic. New York: John Wiley and Sons.

Svarsted, B. L., and Lipton, H. L. 1977. "Informing Parents about Mental Retardation: A Study of Professional Communication and Parent Acceptance." *Social Science and Medicine* 11:645–51.

Sweeney, W. J., and Stern, B. L. 1973. *Woman's Doctor: A Year in the Life of an Obstetrician-Gynecologist.* New York: William Morrow.

Taylor, S. E. 1979. "Hospital Patient Behavior: Reactance, Helplessness, or Control?" *Journal of Social Issues* 35:156–84.

Temin, P. 1980. *Taking Your Medicine: Drug Regulation in the United States.* Cambridge, Mass.: Harvard University Press.

Torgesen, J. K., and Dice, C. 1980. "Characteristics of Research on Learning Disabilities." *Journal of Learning Disabilities* 13:5–9.

Trials of War Criminals before the Nuremberg Military Tribunals under Control Council Law No. 10, Vol. 2. Washington D.C.: U.S. Government Printing Office, 1949.

Tronick, E.; Wise, S.; Als, H.; Adamson, L.; Scanlon, J.; and Brazelton, T. B. 1976. "Regional Obstetric Anesthesia and Newborn

Behavior: Effects over the First Ten Days of Life." *Pediatrics* 58:94–100.

Ucko, L. E. 1965. "A Comparative Study of Asphyxiated and Non-Asphyxiated Boys from Birth to Five Years." *Developmental Medicine and Child Neurology* 7:643–57.

U.S. Bureau of the Census. 1982. *Statistical Abstract of the United States, 1982–83 Edition*. Washington, D.C.: General Printing Office.

U.S. Food and Drug Administration. 1938. Promulgation of Regulations under the Federal Food, Drug, and Cosmetic Act. 3. *Federal Register* 3168, December 28, 1938.

———. 1972. Use of Drugs For Unapproved Indications: Your Legal Responsibility. Washington D.C.

United States Pharmacopoeia Dispensing Information. Part II: For Patients. 1980. Rockville, M.D.: U.S. Pharmacopoeial Convention.

VanderMaelen, A. L.; Strauss, M. E.; and Starr, R. H., Jr. 1975. "Influence of Obstetric Medication on Auditory Habituation in the Newborn." *Developmental Psychology* 11:711–14.

Vorhees, C. V.; Brunner, R. L.; and Butcher, R. E. 1979. "Psychotropic Drugs as Behavioral Teratogens." *Science* 205:1220–25.

Waitzkin, H. 1979. "Medicine, Superstructure and Micropolitics." *Social Science and Medicine* 13A:601–9.

Waitzkin, H., and Stoeckle, J. D. 1976. "Information Control and the Micropolitics of Health Care: Summary of an Ongoing Research Project." *Social Science and Medicine* 10:263–76.

Waitzkin, H., and Waterman, B. 1976. "Social Theory and Medicine." *International Journal of Health Services* 6:9–23.

Wiener, P. C.; Hogg, M. I.; and Rosen, M. 1979. "Neonatal Respiration, Feeding and Neurobehavioral State. Effects of Intrapartum Bupivacaine, Pethidine and Pethidine Reversed by Naloxone." *Anesthesia* 34:996–1004.

Williams, G. M., and Weisburger, J. H. 1983. "Carcinogen Risk Assessment." *Science* 221:6.

Wilson, J. G. 1977. "Current Status of Teratology." In *Handbook of Teratology*. Vol. 1, edited by J. G. Wilson and F. C. Fraser, 47–74. New York: Plenum Press.

Winterscheid, L. C. 1967. "Animal Experimentation Leading to the Development of Advanced Surgical Techniques." *American Journal of Public Health* 57:1604–12.

Woodson, R. H., and DaCosta-Woodson, E. M. 1980. "Covariates of Analgesia in a Clinical Sample and Their Effect on the Relationship between Analgesia and Infant Behavior." *Infant Behavior and Development* 3:205–13.

Woodward, L.; Brackbill, Y.; McManus, K.; Doering, P.; and Robinson, D. 1982. "Exposure to Drugs with Possible Adverse Effects during Pregnancy and Birth." *Birth* 9:165–71.

Wortman, C. B., and Brehm, J. W. 1975. "Responses to Uncontrollable Outcomes: An Integration of Reactance Theory and the Learned Helplessness Model." *Advances in Experimental Social Psychology* 8:278–336.

Writer, W. D. R.; James, F. M.; and Wheeler, A. S. 1981. "Double-Blind Comparison of Morphine and Bupivacaine for Continuous Epidural Analgesia in Labor." *Anesthesiology* 54:215–19.

Yang, R. K.; Zweig, A. R.; Douthitt, T. C.; and Federman, E. J. 1976. "Successive Relationships between Maternal Attitudes during Pregnancy, Analgesic Medication During Labor and Delivery, and Newborn Behavior." *Developmental Psychology* 12:6–14.

Subject Index

Adverse fetal effects. *See* Drug safety

Behavioral teratogenesis, 23–24, 57, 106. *See also* Drugs, obstetric; Drug safety
high-risk period, xxiv–v, 1, 5–6

Center mothers. *See* Florida study, the

Decision making, medical, 25–34, 127. *See also* Disclosure, medical; Informed consent
Demographic variables, 41, 43–46, 96–98, 126
Disclosure, medical, 112–16. *See also* Decision making, medical; Informed consent
and anesthesia, 26
history of, 25–27
information as power, 116–23
to female patients by male physicians, 113, 115, 117, 120–21
Drug administration during childbirth. *See* Drugs, obstetric
Drug consumption, 1
ingredients and products, 137–42

Drug exposure, fetal. *See* Drug safety
Drug information, 2–4, 40, 82, 85–92, 109–15, 123–25. *See also* Disclosure, medical; Drugs, obstetric; Drugs, prenatal; Informed consent
and decision making, 3, 111–12
consumers' right to, 3, 112
correlates of maternal information, 126–27
desire for by consumers, 2–3, 111–12
effects of providing to consumers, 3, 31–33
effects of withholding from consumers, 3, 33–34
Drugs, obstetric, 26. *See also* Drug safety
administration of, 1, 39, 53–57, 59, 61, 78, 101, 137–42
as teratogens, 5–24
effects on infant behaviors, 5–24, 108–9
evaluating seriousness of, 23
general anesthetics, 20–23, 26
information about, 39, 55, 84–85
local anesthetics, 20–21, 23
long-term effects, 23–24
preanesthetics, 20–21, 23

Drugs, prenatal. *See also* Drug
    safety
  consumption of, 1, 38, 49–53,
    61, 78, 99–101, 137–42
  information about, 38–39, 82–
    84, 87–92
Drug safety, 2, 5–24, 57–81,
    101–3. *See also* Drugs, ob-
    stetric; Drugs, prenatal
  animal research, 24, 103–6
  design of research studies, 23,
    107–9
  dosage, 106–7

Florida study, the, 35–103, 126–
    28
Food and Drug Administration
    (FDA), 58–61, 80–81, 102–
    4, 119, 121–25
  congressional intent in legis-
    lating, 122
  policy toward consumers,
    manufacturers, and physi-
    cians, 122–23

Health-promoting behaviors,
    40–41, 93–94, 133–35
Health-related complaints during
    pregnancy, 38, 46–47, 49–
    50, 98

Home mothers. *See* Florida
    study, the
Hospital mothers. *See* Florida
    study, the

Informed consent, 114–15. *See
    also* Decision making, med-
    ical; Disclosure, medical
  ethical values, 27–31
  legal doctrine, 27–31
  respect for autonomy, 28–31
  respect for well-being, 31

Learning disorders
  etiological research, xxiii–v
Locus of Control Scale, 38, 41,
    92–93, 126–27

Medical decision making. *See*
    Decision making, medical

Neonatal Behavioral Assessment
    Scale, 18

Structural teratogenesis, 57, 106
  high-risk period, 1, 5

Teratogenesis. *See* Behavioral
    teratogenesis; Drug safety;
    Structural teratogenesis

Name Index

Alfidi, R. J., 111
Als, H., 15
American Society of Hospital Pharmacists, 38, 82, 85, 95
Applebaum, P. S., 29, 33
Armitage, K. J., 115

Banta, D., 99
Bass, J. W., 32
Bass, R. A., 115
Belsey, E. M., 20
Bertakis, K. D., 32
Bohm, L. C., 33
Bordley, C., 111, 112
Boreham, P., 111, 114
Boyd, J. R., 33
Boyle, J. M., 27, 30, 111, 112, 113, 114
Brackbill, Y., 2, 98, 99, 100
Bradburn, N. M., 42
Brazelton, T. B., 15, 18
Breen, L. J., 41, 126
Brehm, J. W., 34
Brounstein, P. J., 27, 30, 111, 112, 113, 114
Brower, K. R., 19
Brown, N. A., 105
Brown, W. A., 127
Brunner, R. L., xxiv
Butcher, R. E., xxiv
Byrne, T. J., 32

Calvert, E. J., 32, 33
Colcher, I. S., 32

Comstock, L. M., 32
Cranton, J. W., 32
Cruickshank, W. M., xxiii, xxiv

Danziger, S. K., 115, 117
Dice, C., xxiii
Doering, P. L., 1, 99, 100

Eagly, A. H., 120, 121
Egbert, L. D., 32
Ehrenreich, B., 116, 120
Ehrenreich, J., 116, 120
English, D., 120
Ensinck, J. W., 114, 115
Erickson, J. D., 108
Evans, J. W., 41

Fabro, S., 105
Finger, S., 24
Fitzpatrick, R. M., 33
Fleckenstein, L., 111
Frankfort, E., 120
Friedman, C. M., 33
Fuller, S. S., 33

Gaddes, W. H., xxiii
Garber, J., 34
Garfinkel, P., 32
Gibson, D., 111, 114
Gillette, J. L., 32
Goddard, K. E., 108
Gordon, E., 111, 112, 114
Gotsch, A. R., 32, 111

Gray, B. H., 114, 115
Greenspan, R., 33
Grodin, J., 127

Hallahan, D. P., xxiii
Harris, L., 27, 30, 31, 111, 112,
   113, 114
Herman, E., 97
Hill, R. M., 100
Hopkins, A., 33

International Childbirth Educa-
   tion Association, 99
Iseroff, A., 24
Ivy, A. C., 104

Janis, I. L., 32, 33, 34
Joyce, C. R. B., 113

Kanouse, D. E., 32, 111
Kant, I., 28
Kaufmann, C. L., 115, 116
Kennedy, D., 105, 106
Kirke, P. N., 34, 114
Korsch, B. M., 32, 33, 114
Krantz, D. S., 31
Krieser, G., 41
Kron, R. E., 108

Langer, E., 33, 34
Lefcourt, H. M., 41, 126
Lester, B. M., 15, 18
Ley, P., 32, 113
Lidz, C. W., 28, 29, 114
Liguori, S., 32, 111
Lipton, H. L., 114
Lukes, S., 116, 118

McCann, M. B., 105
MacDonald, E. T., 32, 33
MacDonald, J. B., 32, 33
McKenney, J. M., 32

McMahon, F. G., 111
McManus, K. A., 127
Mann, L., 33
Manning, T., 127
Mazis, M., 111, 112, 114
Meisel, A., 28, 29, 114
Mendelsohn, R., 119
Michael, M., 111, 112
Mielke, F., 104
Mikeal, R. L., 32
Milgram, S., 120
Miller, S. M., 117
Miller-Klein, V., 97
Mills, R. T., 31
Mitscherlich, A., 104
Mittleman, F., 33
Miyashita, S., 41
Morris, L. A., 32, 111, 112, 114
Myers, E. D., 32

Negrete, V. F., 32, 33, 114
Norell, S. E., 32

Pardee, G. P., 114, 115
Paulson, P. T., 33
Pernick, M. S., 25, 26
Phares, E. J., 126
Phoenix, M., 32, 33
Pohl, J. M., 33
President's Commission for the
   Study of Ethical Problems in
   Medicine and Biomedical and
   Behavioral Research, 3, 27,
   29, 30, 31, 111, 113, 115
Price, J. L. W., 33
Prociuk, T. J., 41, 126
PsyINFO Retrospective, xxiii
Puretz, J., 24
Putt, A. M., 32

Rice, J., 2, 98, 99
Robinson, H. J., 105

Rodin, J., 33, 34
Roncari, I., 32
Rosenberg, S. G., 113
Ross, D. M., xxiv
Ross, S. A., xxiv
Roth, L. H., 28, 29, 33
Rotter, J. B., 38, 41, 92
Russo, E. J., 41
Ruzek, S., 113
Ryan, J., 111

Saunderson, G. R., 32
Schneiderman, L. J., 115
Schultz, A. L., 114, 115
Schulz, R., 33
Seeman, M., 41
Seligman, M. E. P., 33, 34, 117
Seltzer, A., 32
Shapiro, M. C., 111, 115, 117
Sharpe, T. R., 32
Shaw, N. S., 33
Simons, D., 24
Spelman, M. S., 113
Stare, F. J., 105
Starr, P., 118, 121
Stein, M., 108
Stern, B. L., 113
Stewart, R. B., 1, 100
Stoeckle, J. D., 41, 114
Sudman, S., 42

Surgeon General's Advisory
    Committee on Smoking and
    Health, 107, 109
Svarsted, B. L., 32, 114
Sweeney, W. J., 113

Taylor, S. E., 34
Temin, P., 122
Thacker, S., 99
Torgesen, J. K., xxiii

Ucko, L. E., 23
U.S. Bureau of the Census, 96
U.S. Food and Drug Adminis-
    tration, 119, 122

Ventre, F., 97
Vorhees, C. V., xxiv

Wack, J. T., 33
Waitzkin, H., 41, 114, 116, 119
Waterman, B., 116
Weisburger, J. H., 106
Williams, G. M., 106
Wilson, J. G., 5, 106
Wine, J., 41, 126
Winterscheid, L. C., 105
Woodward, L., 100
Wortman, C. B., 34

Young, D., 2, 98, 99

www.ingramcontent.com/pod-product-compliance
Lightning Source LLC
Chambersburg PA
CBHW020351270326
41926CB00007B/395